Acupuncture

& IVF

D1566680

Tredyffrin Public Library
582 Upper Gulph Road
Strafford, PA 19087
(610) 688-7092

Acupuncture & IVF

Dr. Lifang Liang

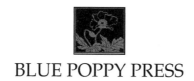

BLUE POPPY PRESS

Published by:
BLUE POPPY PRESS
A Division of Blue Poppy Enterprises, Inc.
5441 Western Ave., Suite 2
BOULDER, CO 80301

First Edition, August 2003
Second Printing, March 2004
Third Printing, February 2005

ISBN 1-891845-24-1
LCCN #2003108251

COPYRIGHT © BLUE POPPY PRESS, 2003. All Rights Reserved.

All rights reserved. No part of this book may be reproduced, stored in a
retrieval system, transcribed in any form or by any means, electronic,
mechanical, photocopy, recording, or any other means, or translated into any
language without the prior written permission of the publisher.

DISCLAIMER: The information in this book is given in good faith.
However, the author and the publishers cannot be held responsible for
any error or omission. The publishers will not accept liabilities for any
injuries or damages caused to the reader that may result from the reader's
acting upon or using the content contained in this book. The publishers
make this information available to English language readers for
research and scholarly purposes only.

The publishers do not advocate nor endorse self-medication by laypersons.
Chinese medicine is a professional medicine. Laypersons interested in avail-
ing themselves of the treatments described in this book should seek out a
qualified professional practitioner of Chinese medicine.

COMP Designation: Original work using a standard translational terminology

10 9 8 7 6 5 4 3

Printed at Victor Graphics, Inc., Baltimore, MD

Testimonials & Endorsements
for Dr. Liang & this Book

As I finally sat down at 9:40 P.M. trying to write this foreword for Dr. Liang's book on her work with acupuncture and herbs to enhance fertility and wondered where should I begin, my precious daughter woke up in the next room calling for "Mommy." Oh, her sweet little voice makes me rush over to her anytime day and night. Sometimes our little princess decides that she had enough sleep and wants to get up and play at 4:30 A.M.—and I will be her playmate. But how did I get to be the mother of this sweet and beautiful little girl? It was a long, five-year journey.

My husband and I got married in 1995. After a year and a half, when I was 33 and my husband, Hal, was 37, we started trying to get pregnant, thinking that we were at the best point in our relationship to have a child. Hal warned me during our three year courtship that he has a condition called varicocele that is associated with infertility. A varicocele is a common structural abnormality in the vascular system within the scrotal sac that can affect sperm quality. However, many men with a varicocele have normal fertility. I did not gave it too much thought at the time. We attempted conception without medical assistance for three months and nothing happened. Tests then showed that my husband had a low sperm count. Our doctor at the time said that, with his sperm count, we should proceed to intrauterine insemination (IUI).

So we started our journey of infertility treatment. My husband underwent a high tech radiological treatment that cured the varicocele but did not increase his sperm count. I went though nine IUIs with or without medications in two years. I was on an emotional roller coaster every time. I was having a hard time even talking to my friends who just had a baby or to relatives at holiday get-togethers. Then we took the next step and went on to *in vitro* fertilization (IVF). Through IVF, I produced eight eggs—a disturbingly low number for a 35 year-old woman pumped full of synthetic hormones. I was labeled a "low responder." The eggs were then fertilized with my husband's sperm and four embryos developed and were placed in my uterus. I did not get pregnant. I was very disappointed and sad. My husband and I went on to get some group counseling and, during the session, I mentioned that I was not getting my period and was thinking this was probably do to the effect of the fertility drugs. The therapist advised us to get checked. We had the beta HCG tested. To our surprise, the number came out positive and was quite high. My husband and I were overjoyed that we actually conceived on our own, but I started bleeding the following morning—I miscarried.

I did not have any courage to try IVF again until a year later, after we moved to the Bay area due to my husband's job change. We thought we should give Stanford IVF program a try since we live only 20 minutes from the medical center. This second IVF was another big disappointment. This time I produced even less eggs—six eggs, four fertilized, and three developed embryos. I did not get pregnant. I was devastated. I was not sure if I could take any more disappointment. My husband and I started talking about adoption. It was at this point that a family friend suggested that we give acupuncture a try.

With reluctance I started doing some more research to educate myself first. I searched the Internet and found an article on www.acupuncture.com, "Chinese Medicine and Assisted Reproductive Technology for the Modern Couple." I decided that I couldn't go through another negative cycle of IVF emotionally without strengthening and balancing my own body. I contacted the author of the article for a referral in the San Francisco Bay area. Dr. Liang's name was given to me. My husband was very skeptical about traditional Chinese medicine, since he himself was trained in Western medicine. But with my persuasion, he finally agreed too try a few sessions of acupuncture and take the herbal medicine for the sake of making me happy.

I regarded the herbs as a final hope and I felt that the herbs might contain beneficial ingredients that had escaped the detection of Western medicine. My husband, on the other hand, was very skeptical of the herbs and called them "those awful roots and twigs." With great reluctance, he would slowly sip his herbs each evening under my watchful gaze. Likewise, I gladly accepted acupuncture as a means to change my body, to alter my physiology in ways that would promote conception. To my surprise, my husband found acupuncture very relaxing and developed a warm rapport with Dr. Liang.

After nine months of treatment with Dr. Liang and with great trepidation, I underwent IVF for a third time at Stanford. We agreed before that this would be our final attempt. This round yielded five fertilized eggs and developed four embryos. All four were implanted and then we waited. With guarded glee we learned that I was pregnant again. I continued the herbs for the nail-biting first trimester. I was frightened by a small amount of bleeding that my husband did not tell me is associated with miscarriage. Once I reached the second trimester I could relax somewhat. I knew that the odds were in our favor and that we would soon be parents.

As I cuddle my little girl to sleep and inhale her sweet scent every time, watching our little girl with her giggles and smiles, I feel very lucky and effusively thankful of the help that Dr. Liang gave us. We received the best that Western medicine has to offer from top physicians at the most prestigious medical centers in California and did not have a child until we received traditional Chinese medical treatment from Dr. Liang. My husband, the physician, believes that Chinese medicine is only a placebo, but I do not care because it worked for us and we are very, very happy.

Jenny Morrison

I first had the privilege of meeting Dr. Li-fang Liang in 1990 when I began my studies at the American College of Traditional Chinese Medicine (ACTCM). I had the good fortune to be a student of Dr. Liang's throughout my training, both in the classroom and in the clinic. From this magnificent teacher, I had the opportunity to learn the full spectrum of Chinese medicine—from the basic foundations to classical theory—and the full range of clinical skills, including patient intake, acupuncture protocols, and perhaps most significantly, herbal formulas, of which Dr. Liang is a master. Dr. Liang gave me the skills and knowledge I required to successfully begin my own medical career specializing in women's health and fertility. This book is written to bring her knowledge to a wider audience, including acupuncturists, students, and Western M.D.s.

Dr. Liang began her own medical career over 30 years ago in China where she was trained as both an M.D. and an acupuncturist and herbalist, specializing in women's health and fertility. Almost from the beginning, Dr. Liang recognized the challenges many couples faced in conceiving children and felt that the low success rates of various fertility treatments could be much improved, particularly through the integration of Eastern and Western medicine. She made the research and application of this integration her lifelong work. In 1989, she came to the U.S., where she spent one year researching fertility at a major Western medical university. In 1990, she relocated to San Francisco where she joined the faculty at ACTCM and established her private practice. Over the last 10 years, Dr. Liang has thoroughly researched the many benefits of combining Chinese medicine with Western medically assisted reproductive technologies, particularly *in vitro* fertilization (IVF). This book is based on those many years of research and Dr. Liang's experience in helping to increase the success rates of IVF.

Specifically, this book examines the use of traditional Chinese medicine before, during, and after the IVF cycle. Dr. Liang explains how the 2-3 months prior to an IVF cycle can be best spent preparing the system for the IVF procedure. During the IVF cycle itself, Chinese medicine can help increase the number of follicles and improve the quality of the uterine environment. Once pregnant, Chinese medicine can be helpful in preventing unnecessary miscarriages. Dr. Liang thoroughly discusses the combination of acupuncture and Chinese medicinals, bringing great insight into the formulas and modifications she recommends with her many years of clinical experience.

Dr. Liang hopes that this text will edify both acupuncturists and M.D.s alike. The acupuncturist will acquire valuable information to better assist their fertility patients in the clinic, while the M.D. will gain a deeper understanding of how Chinese medicine can be effectively incorporated into IVF protocols with great benefit to the patient due to a significant increase in success rates. This cross pollination of medical knowledge results in an integrated approach that takes the best of what both systems have to offer and provides the patient with the maximum chance for success.

Leslie Oldershaw, L.Ac.

Western medicine has traditionally been resistant to alternative therapies, instead focusing on the management of disease after it presents, often ignoring the fact that a particular organ or system actually belongs to a person or patient. Alternative therapies and traditional medicine in many cultures have focused on the whole person and have generally asked the questions about causation and methods of prevention. Ignoring lifestyle, diet, exercise, and the power of the mind, practitioners of Western medicine have forced patients to choose between Western medicine and alternative therapies instead of combining the best of both worlds.

Dr. Lifang Liang, a physician and a healer, has been trained in both Chinese and Western medicines, with special emphasis in gynecology. For 14 years as an assistant professor in China, Dr. Liang taught Chinese medicine while performing surgery and applying the techniques of Western medicine in her practice. In March of 1989, she moved to the University of Texas Medical School in San Antonio. True to her training, Dr. Liang wanted to incorporate the complementary modalities of Chinese medicine and Western medicine but, due to bureaucratic roadblocks, this was not permitted. San Antonio's loss became San Francisco's gain, and Dr. Liang joined the faculty of the American College of Traditional Chinese Medicine (ACTCM).

In this book, Dr. Liang shares with us many intensely personal, life-altering events, including the loss of her mother at age nine and the impact that this had on directing her to become a healer and nurturer rather than an engineer. The epiphany for her was the almost miraculous improvement of a patient with intracranial tuberculosis when Chinese medicine was added to conventional Western medical therapy during her internship.

Practitioners of Western medicine have long been skeptical about alternative therapies, mainly out of ignorance of the exact nature of the theory and the practice and also out of fear of competition and possible loss of livelihood. Dr. Liang very eloquently outlines the complementary nature of the Eastern and the Western approach and explains in detail the concepts of the yin and yang, the vital substances of qi, blood, essence, and body fluids along with the five phases and their interaction. In this book, she provides a means for Westerners, both medical practitioners and patients, of understanding the basis of therapies that have evolved over more than 4,000 years in China, while also providing details of acupuncture and herbal therapies which will enable other practitioners of Chinese medicine to compare protocols and communicate and collaborate to further improve outcomes.

Christo Zouves, M.D.
Medical Director, Zouves Fertility Center
Author: "Expecting Miracles"

I am honored to have the opportunity to present Dr. Li-fang Liang's book, *Acupuncture & IVF*. Infertility and the use of assisted reproductive techniques (ART) are becoming more prevalent over time. Despite an overall increase in access to healthcare, infertility rates for women continue to increase. Popular explanations include delayed average age of child-bearing attempts and changing social and economic roles for women which, in turn, lead to delayed or alternative fertility plans.

Many women ultimately consider *in vitro* fertilization in their attempts to start a family. Until very recently, most *in vitro* fertilization centers utilized a Western medical approach exclusively. Fortunately, Dr. Li-fang Liang and other Chinese medical specialists have been able to demonstrate how one's chances of having a successful and healthy pregnancy can be maximized by combining Western medicine with Chinese medicine. This holistic view and team approach to tackle the obstacle of infertility brings "the best of both worlds" strategy to a formidable problem.

Dr. Liang's extensive experience with infertility patients and unique training in both Western and Chinese medicine combine in this book to provide practitioners and patients with a comprehensive and effective plan for a successful IVF cycle.

Katherine T. Hsiao, M.D., F.A.C.O.G.

Having gone through three failed years of infertility treatments—four IUIs and two IVFs—I chose to spend a year in acupuncture since I had heard it might help. Ever since I stopped taking birth control pills three years ago, my natural menstrual cycles never returned and the doctors told me they probably never would. They said pregnancy would require fertility treatments. While sitting in the waiting area of my fertility doctor, a woman mentioned her success with Dr. Li-fang Liang and acupuncture in her efforts to get pregnant. Once I had confirmed my last IVF had not worked, I made an appointment with Dr. Liang. Within four weeks of weekly acupuncture treatments and daily herbs, I had my first menstrual cycle. And they continued every month from that time forward. As I charted my cycles and continued the weekly appointments and daily herbs, I definitely felt my body changing and becoming more "normal." After nine months of treatment, I discovered I was pregnant—a condition my fertility doctor never thought I would achieve naturally. I continued to see Dr. Liang for treatments and herbs for the first 30 weeks of my pregnancy and can happily report that, within the next few weeks, my husband and I will welcome the birth of our first child! I highly recommend anyone struggling with infertility to consider acupuncture. It made all the difference in the world for me!

Kristin Kennedy

Acknowledgements

I acknowledge with sincere gratitude the many people who have, in one way or another, helped me in writing this book.

The most important period of my professional training was spent at the Guangzhou University of Chinese Medicine in China, and, in the U.S.A., at the University of Texas Medical School and the American Global University. I am deeply indebted to these institutions' directors and teachers as well as other staff members for their care and patience in sharing their profound knowledge with me.

Furthermore, I am greatly indebted to my professor, the late Dr. Huanshen Wu for sharing his 40 years of clinical experience in treating infertility with me.

I would also like to thank Robert Schenken, M.D., of the University of Texas Medical School for training me in IVF techniques.

I would like to express my appreciation to the following Western physicians for their support and help, especially Dr. Katherine T. Hsiao, Dr. Christo Zouves, Dr. Victor Y. Fujimoto, and Dr. Phillip Chenette.

I would especially like to thank my students, Adriel Breault, Suzanne Delbou, Jennifer Everett, Johanna B. Flynn, Debra Sue Kelvin, Heidi Kirkpatrick, Faye H. Luong, Elisa Overholt, Diane Tuet, and Anne Wees from the American College of Traditional Chinese Medicine for their interest in learning from me and their assistance in creating this book. Thank you also to my patients for lending their assistance and giving me useful feedback in my effort of writing this book.

Acknowledgements

Finally, I could not have accomplished this work without the constant support and inspiration of my loving husband, Mr. Yiwang Xie. I am also very appreciative of my son, Min Xie, for helping me to write this book even though he was busy with his studies at Stanford University.

Lifang Liang, O.M.D., Ph.D., L.Ac.

Preface

My name is Lifang Liang. I am a Chinese medical doctor. While living in China, I was a student of both Chinese and Western medicine. I studied at Guangzhou University of Chinese Medicine for six years. After graduation, I was selected to work at the same school as a doctor and an assistant professor. I spent an additional six years receiving an advanced education in gynecology in both Western medicine and Chinese medicine. For 14 years, I taught in the Chinese medical school, performed surgeries in the hospital, and practiced acupuncture, herbal medicine, and Western medicine.

In March of 1989, the University of Texas Medical School in San Antonio invited me to the United States to conduct Western medical research on *in vitro* fertilization (IVF) with DNA and RNA assays. The experience was valuable, but my primary interest was in Chinese medical research. Many doctors asked, "Why are you interested in Chinese medicine?" This question caused me to think deeply. In addition, for the first five years in America, I was separated from my husband and son who were still in China. I missed them very much. At times I felt so lonely and asked myself why I came to the United States.

Upon reflection, the answer was rooted in my past. As a child when I was studying in school, I liked mathematics very much and dreamed of being an engineer. However, my family was poor and my mother died when I was nine years old. This event altered my mind. I did not want children to suffer from the loss of their mother's care. Therefore, I decided to become a doctor to help people. So I went to medical school. First, I was very excited, but soon I felt tired because I needed to memorize more than one thousand herbs and hundreds of acupuncture points and many medical theories. I almost wanted to stop learning Chinese medicine.

My true belief in Chinese medicine began when I was an intern in the hospital working with a patient who suffered from brain tuberculosis that resulted in partial paralysis. He was unable to move his left arm and leg and he lay in bed for six months. I used acupuncture needles on some points with strong stimulation for five treatments. When I came to the ward to treat him again, I could not find the patient in bed. "Li Shan! Where are you?" I called loudly. "I am here!" he responded unseen. Following the sound, I found the patient. I could not believe my eyes! He was standing in line for supper. "Who has brought you here?" I asked very surprised. He was very happy to tell me, "I can walk slowly along the wall." After that, he was given acupuncture 10 more times. Consequently, he could walk normally and even jump. Finally he recovered completely and left the hospital. Since then I have realized the power of Chinese medicine in treating disease, thus solidifying my commitment to its practice.

In China, Western medicine is combined with Chinese medicine in most hospitals and medical schools. For some diseases, Chinese medicine is used all by itself. For others, the use of Western medicine or surgery is the preferred option. Many diseases benefit from using both modalities at the same time and this approach had garnered more positive results than either medicine alone. I believe in both Chinese and Western medicine—each have their strengths and weaknesses. Their strengths compliment each other and it is my experience that, when judiciously employed, they can correct each other's weaknesses. In China, we believe that two hands are better than one. Similarly, when it comes to medicine, I believe two methods are better than only one method.

Therefore, I wanted to incorporate both modalities in San Antonio, but the medical school could not accommodate this request. Herbs were not permitted and there were no research funds for this purpose. Meanwhile, the American College of Traditional Chinese Medicine (ACTCM) invited me to come to San Francisco. By that time, my research to improve semen motility was already successful. My co-workers warned, "Don't go to San Francisco; they have earthquakes."

This tactic did not deter me!

I accepted the offer from ACTCM and went to San Francisco in 1989 to offer my experience in Chinese medicine (the same year San Francisco had its big earthquake). Since then, I have been a professor at ACTCM as well as treat patients in a private practice at the 450 Sutter Medical Building. Additionally, I recently completed a Ph.D. in advanced research in the treatment of infertility with Chinese and Western medicines from the American Global University Program for Oriental Medical Research. I work with Western infertility specialists and, by combining the benefits of both Chinese and Western medicines, we have increased the success rate of IVF with our patients. Now I would like to share my experience.

Often, I have found the translation of Chinese medicine books into English were not always correct. I made up my mind to improve my English language skills with the hopes that, in the future, I could translate or write better Chinese medical books in English. In so doing, my wish is to expand the world's knowledge of Chinese medicine and to help improve medicine worldwide.

Table of Contents

Introduction

There are many different ways to get to one goal. Both Chinese and Western medicines have accomplished great feats over the last century, treating numerous diseases, saving thousands of lives, and improving the quality of life for countless others. Using the best of both worlds, it is my experience that it is possible to increase the success rate of *in vitro* fertilization significantly.

In fact, a recent German study found that using acupuncture with IVF achieved a 42% clinical pregnancy rate in the test group, compared to 26% in the control group that did not receive acupuncture. This study involved giving acupuncture for just one day, shortly before and after the transfer of embryos. My clinical experience is that this rate increases to at least 60% with broader support of both Chinese herbs and acupuncture in preparation for and support throughout the IVF procedure. As well, both of these modalities can significantly reduce the risk of miscarriage by supporting the female during her entire pregnancy.

A large number of patients who have tried IVF several times and were unsuccessful have soon become pregnant after Chinese medicine treatments. In clinical observation, the ultrasound shows that, after acupuncture, the color of women's ovaries change from cloudy to bright and clear. The follicles usually double in number, the lining of the uterus becomes thicker, and the number of embryos increases significantly. Patients experience less side effects from the Western drugs and feel more at ease and happy. For male patients, it is my experience that the semen quality significantly improves and the sperm number greatly increases. In brief, Chinese medicine can help to improve the success rate of IVF in a number of ways:

1. Improve the function of the ovaries to produce better quality eggs
2. Regulate the hormones to produce a larger number of follicles
3. Increase blood flow to the uterus and increase the thickness of the uterine lining
4. Relax the patient and decrease their stress
5. Prevent the uterus from contracting
6. Lessen the side effects of drugs used in IVF
7. Strengthen the immune system
8. Improve semen to create better quality and quantity of embryos
9. Decrease chances of miscarriage

The goal of this book is to share the formula and point combinations that I have found to be the most clinically successful for IVF. In addition, traditional formulas for infertility are referenced for historical perspective and further understanding.

A note on formulas & dosages

In Chinese, *fang* is a general term meaning "formula." A formula or *fang* can be prepared as a *tang*, a decoction from bulk-dispensed medicinals, as a *san* or powdered prescription, or as *wan* or pills. In my practice, I primarily prescribe my formulas as decoctions or powders, although I also sometimes use ready-made pills.

Through my years of experience, I have developed several of my own formulas. For these, I have used the term *fang* instead of the more commonly used *tang* since it is up to the individual practitioner to decide whether to prescribe these formulas as decoctions, powders, or pills based on the particular needs and wishes of each patient. Further, because my name (Lifang) includes a homonym of the word *fang*, it has a special meaning for me in terms of the formulas I myself have created.

As readers will note, I have not provided dosages for the formulas in this text as they will vary depending on the patient's condition as well as with the method of preparation and administration. However, to help those new to the prescription of Chinese medicinals, a general range has been provided for individual medicinals which are used in the various formulas discussed in this book. Appendices have also been provided listing important Western drugs and Chinese herbal medicinals which are useful in addressing reproductive issues.

1

Overview of Chinese Medicine

Chinese medicine (*zhong yi*) is an ancient healing art that has been practiced in China for more than 4,000 years. Acupuncture, the most commonly used modality of Chinese medicine in the West, utilizes sterilized needles to access a person's qi or "vital energy." The needles are placed in points found along the channels that run throughout the entire body. The channels are connected to internal organs as well as to the exterior body. Acupuncture rectifies and harmonizes the body's energy and expels pathogenic factors. It can strengthen the immune system, enhance circulation, regulate hormones, increase energy, and reduce stress. Other treatment modalities include herbal therapy, dietary recommendations, massage, and lifestyle counseling.

Chinese medicine came about from many years of observing nature and the cycle of life. Its theories are based upon yin and yang, vital substances, and the five phases. Many texts are available in English that discuss these topics extensively. However, for the purposes of this book, a brief overview of Chinese medical theory will be provided, especially as it relates to infertility.

Yin & yang

Chinese yin-yang theory is the basis of Chinese medicine. Yin-yang theory is a kind of philosophical dualism. According to this theory, everything in the phenomenal world has yin and yang aspects. Yin and yang are inseparable, interchangeable, mutually creating, and transforming. Yin represents such things as night, cold, substance, and the interior, while yang appears as day, heat, activity, and the exterior. Although we can say that this is more yin relative to that being more yang, in fact, yin and yang are mutually rooted and mutually engendering. In Chinese medicine, different parts and functions of the body are yin as compared to other parts and functions being yang.

Vital substances

The vital substances of Chinese medicine include qi, blood (*xue*), essence (*jing*), and body fluids (*jin ye*). Qi represents one's "life force" or "vital energy," while blood is the nutrition that constructs and sustains the body. Similar to yin and yang, qi and blood have an extremely close relationship. Qi engenders and transforms the blood, but blood is the mother of the qi. Qi pushes the blood through the body, while blood carries qi along with it. It is said that heaven and earth are yang and yin in the outside world, but that qi and blood are yang and yin respectively in the human body. Any form of vacuity or repletion of yin, yang, qi, or blood may result in pain, dysfunction, or disease.

There are three types of essence. Former heaven essence (sometimes called prenatal essence in English) is derived from the parents and provides for a person's constitutional make-up. It is a fixed substance that cannot be added to or replenished. Latter heaven essence (a.k.a. postnatal or acquired essence) is a general term that describes the essence that is derived after birth from food, air, and fluids. Both pre- and postnatal essences contribute to kidney essence which is responsible for growth, development, sexual maturation, reproduction, and pregnancy. This essence is referred to as the root of life and provides for our basic constitutional strength.

The five phases

In five phase (*wu xing*) theory, each phase corresponds to a seasonal time in nature and to a yin and yang organ in the body. Yin viscera store vital substances (qi, blood, essence, and body fluids), while their paired yang bowels receive, transform, and course the vital substances. Unlike Western medicine, which tends to focus on an organ's material and functional qualities, Chinese medicine sees each organ as part of a larger complex that includes not only those tangible aspects but encompasses other associations as well, such as emotion, color, and taste (see figure 1).

	Wood	Fire	Earth	Metal	Water
Yin Organ	Liver	Heart	Spleen	Lung	Kidney
Yang Organ	Gallbladder	Small Intestine	Stomach	Large Intestine	Urinary Bladder
Season	Spring	Summer	Late Summer	Autumn	Winter
Color	Green	Red	Yellow	White	Black
Taste	Sour	Bitter	Sweet	Acrid	Salty
Development	Birth	Growth	Transformation	Harvest	Storage
Tissues	Sinews	Vessels	Muscles	Skin	Bones
Affects	Anger	Joy	Thought	Sadness	Fear

Figure 1.

In relation to Western medicine, the functional qualities of internal organs in Chinese medicine often overlap. For example, in Chinese medicine, the heart includes the spirit or mental system, but, similar to Western medicine, it also helps circulate the blood. The lungs include the respiratory system and also help "govern" the qi of the entire body. The endocrine system in Western medicine is recognized as part of the kidneys' function in Chinese medicine. The kidneys are also responsible for growth, development, and reproduction. In addition to storing blood, the liver regulates the emotions and the flow of qi. Lastly, the spleen represents the digestive system and the body's ability to transform and transport the nutrients received from food and drink.

The five phases are interlinked to one another. Each phase is generated by another but also held in check by a third. For example, the heart is generated by the liver (see figure 2) but controlled by the kidney (see figure 3).

When one phase falls out of balance, the others are easily affected. An imbalance can allow pathologies to occur, resulting in disease.

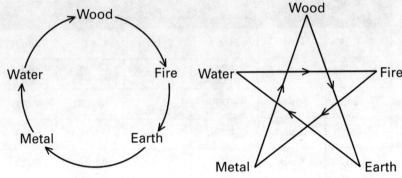

Figure 2. Generating Cycle   **Figure 3**. Controlling Cycle

The six evils

There are six species of pathological energy (*liu xie*) in Chinese medicine. These are referred to as evil qi and include dampness, heat, cold, wind, dryness, and summerheat. If any of these energies or types of qi are either insufficient or excessive, whether inside the body or out, they can cause disease.

Dampness

In relation to nature, dampness is represented by rain and fog and can be explained in medical theory as excessive fluid accumulation in the body. Gynecological conditions often associated with damp evils include ovarian cysts, leukorrhea, and frequent vaginal infections.

Heat

Heat can be either replete or vacuous in nature, showing up as a fast metabolism, anxiety, or hyperactivity accompanied by heat symptoms such as hot flashes and/or night sweats. Accompanied by dampness, heat may also and often does correspond to infection by pathogens such as bacteria and viruses.

Cold

Cold can be of a replete or vacuous nature, thereby slowing metabolism. Cold can cause lethargy and dysmenorrhea with a feeling of cold in the abdomen that is relieved by warmth.

Wind

Wind can invade the body as an externally contracted pathogen, such as a bacteria or virus. In relation to gynecological disorders, there may also be internal wind caused by severe imbalance of the body's yin, yang, qi, or blood and leading to symptoms of vertigo, headaches, and possibly fainting.

Dryness

Dryness causes or is caused by a depletion of the body's yin fluids. Therefore, dryness can result in drying of vaginal fluids and other symptoms associated with menopause.

Summerheat

While the previous five evils can all have either internal or external species, summerheat can only be an externally contracted evil. Summerheat refers to externally contracted dampness and heat in the summer and early fall in hot, damp climates. Happily for our purposes, summerheat does not play much of a role in Chinese gynecology.

The viscera & bowels

There are five viscera (*zang*) and six bowels (*fu*) in Chinese medicine. The five viscera include the liver, heart, lungs, spleen, and kidneys. The six bowels are the stomach, small intestine, large intestine, gallbladder, bladder, and triple burner. This last "bowel" refers to the chest, upper, and lower abdomen and the coordinated functioning of the other viscera and bowels located in these three areas of the torso. In addition, there are six extraordinary bowels. These are extraordinary or unique because they do not participate in the yin-yang and five phase paired relationships of the preceding viscera and bowels. They are also extraordinary because, although they are hollow in form, they store essence. These six extraordinary bowels include the brain, spinal cord, gallbladder, uterus, bones, and blood vessels. However, the three main viscera related to female reproduction in Chinese medicine are the kidneys, spleen, and liver.

The kidneys

In addition to storing the essence, the kidneys have two aspects: kidney yin which provides substance, and kidney yang which provides force. Both are very important factors of the female reproductive system. A vacuity of kidney yin, resulting from overwork, a long, chronic disease, or too many children born too close together, leads to a drying up of yin and, therefore, the cessation of the menses. *Yi Xue Zheng Chuan (The Correct Transmission of the Study of Medicine)* refers to this depletion of kidney yin saying, "The menses are a transformation of kidney water; when this is vacuous, menstrual blood dries up." Kidney yang vacuity may lead to the formation of cold which obstructs the uterus and may cause infertility.

Kidney essence is the origin of menstrual blood which has many functions in Chinese medicine. Blood flows throughout the body sending nutrients to every cell and supplying the woman's menstrual cycle. Once pregnancy has occurred, blood nourishes the embryo's growth. When the child is born, blood turns into the mother's milk and supplies the infant with nourishment.

The spleen

The spleen has several important functions. The spleen transforms and transports food and drink and sends the clear qi out to the entire body and the turbid qi down and out through the intestines. The spleen also forms blood which is very important to a woman's menstrual cycle. If the spleen qi is vacuous, it is not able to make enough blood, and the woman may experience delayed and/or scanty menstruation or amenorrhea. The spleen also has the function of holding the blood within the vessels. If the spleen fails to manage or contain the blood, there may be spotting or heavy uterine bleeding.

The liver

According to Chinese medical theory, the liver plays a very important role in the reproductive systems in both men and women. The liver governs the free coursing of qi throughout the entire body and it stores blood at night. Since the qi moves the blood, if the qi stops, the blood stops. This means that, if the qi becomes stagnant, the blood may eventually become static. Qi stagnation and blood stasis often go hand in hand and cause such problems as endometriosis, uterine fibroids, and ovarian cysts. Often, qi stagnation and blood stasis may present with symptoms of abdominal pain, cramps, or irregular menstruation. In men, this blockage of qi and blood may manifest as varicoceles or obstruction of the ejaculatory ducts. High levels of stress impede the free flow of qi and, thus, often cause binding depression of liver qi. If there is liver blood vacuity, there may be scanty menstruation, dizziness, headaches, and problems with fertility.

The channels & network vessels

Each of the viscera and bowels of Chinese medicine has an associated channel (*jing*) and various network vessels (*luo*) that run along specific pathways on the body and can be accessed through the acupuncture points. These are referred to as the regular channels (*zheng jing*). In addition, the body has several extraordinary vessels (*qi mai*) that act as reservoirs to these regular channels. These extraordinary vessels can both hold replete qi from the main channels as well as give qi back to them as needed. In gynecology, two of the most important of these eight extraordinary vessels are the controlling (*ren*) and thoroughfare (*chong*) vessels. The controlling vessel, also known as the "sea of yin," helps regulate menstruation, fertility, conception, pregnancy, childbirth, and menopause. Often referred to as the "sea of blood," the thoroughfare vessel nourishes the blood and works in concert with the controlling vessel to regulate the uterus and menstruation. Both of these vessels derive their qi from the kidneys and help circulate kidney essence throughout the body. The girdling vessel (*dai mai*) is the only horizontal channel of the body. It influences the genitals and is thought to have a containing function, encircling the other channels.

The *tian gui* or heavenly water

The *Huang Di Nei Jing (Yellow Emperor's Inner Classic)*, first completed approximately 2,500 years ago, is one of the most fundamental pieces of Chinese medical literature. It describes a woman's physiological changes in seven year increments having to do with the waxing and waning of something called the *tian gui* or heavenly water. The heavenly water refers to kidney essence in its role in creating the menstruate. Therefore, menarche is called "the arrival of the *tian gui*", while menopause is called "the cessation of the *tian gui*." For example, at two times seven or 14 years of age, a girl's kidney essence has developed and, therefore, her menstruation starts and she is able to conceive. At three times seven or 21, her kidney essence has optimized and she is ready for conception. At five times seven or 35, a woman's kidney essence has begun to wane, and by age 42, it is rapidly diminishing. At seven times seven or 49 years of age, the woman's kidney essence is now depleted and, therefore, her menstruation stops and she can no longer conceive.

This classical theory describes the normal physiology of a woman's hormonal cycle throughout her life. Due to the cultural difference and the improvement in both nutrition and living environment, modern women in North America and Europe on average start their puberty 1-3 years earlier and enter their menopause 2-3 years later than those living in ancient times. In spite of this slight difference between ancient and modern-day women, the basic ideas about the physiology of female menstruation in the *Huang Di Nei Jing* are still an important guide to modern traditional Chinese medical diagnosis and its treatment of gynecological diseases.

2

The Pathology of Infertility

Western medical pathologies of female reproduction

There are several primary pathological conditions that may interfere with a female's ability to achieve pregnancy:

1. Ovarian factors

At around 41 years of age, the function of a woman's ovaries starts to decline. (Although this is a natural stage of a woman's development, for the purposes of achieving pregnancy, it is considered a pathology here.) This decline results in the production of lesser quality eggs. Fertilization of these eggs is more difficult and, generally, they do not develop as well after fertilization. When the ovaries decline in function, follicle-stimulating hormone (FSH) levels increase in order to induce ovulation. FSH levels above 10 indicate that the ovarian function has declined, making pregnancy more difficult to achieve. Even when pregnancy does occur, it is usually more difficult for the woman to carry the embryo to term, and miscarriage often results. In addition, estrogen and progesterone levels decrease, causing a thinning of the endometrium. All of these factors affect the implantation of the embryo.

Another condition of the ovaries is the occasional or total failure to ovulate. This may be due to hormonal changes causing irregular menstruation, amenorrhea, or heavy uterine bleeding. This condition may also be due to polycystic ovaries.

The treatment for these conditions focuses on regulating the menses, balancing hormone levels, and if needed, treating polycysts and endometriosis. Once this is achieved, fertility is greatly increased.

2. Fallopian tube factors

The fallopian tubes may become blocked due to infection or endometriosis causing adhesions. As a result, the sperm is unable to fertilize the egg.

3. Uterine factors

Uterine (fibroid) myomas distort the uterine cavity or block the interstitial parts of the tubes, thus preventing the embryo from moving to the uterus. Another problem arises when the uterus is too small for the embryo to grow and develop.

4. Cervical factors

Cervical or vaginal infection can cause repletion discharge or mucus which may kill or inhibit the advance of the sperm. This may be due to the presence of antibodies.

Female pathology according to Chinese medicine

In order for fertilization to occur, the yin, yang, qi, and blood of the kidneys all need to be perfectly balanced. When one or more of these elements is out of balance, a disharmony results and infertility may occur. When diagnosing infertility, it is important to differentiate clearly between cases of vacuity and cases of repletion. The following patterns relate to the uterus and the thoroughfare and controlling vessels, which include the ovaries and fallopian tubes.

1. Vacuity patterns

A. Blood & yin vacuity

If the liver blood and kidney yin are vacuous, the essence will not be sufficient to nourish the uterus and the thoroughfare and controlling vessels. This condition may bring about various problems with the eggs, such as the inability of the egg to be fertilized, the fertilized egg not being able to implant itself and grow, or the lack of any eggs.

B. Qi & yang vacuity

When there is a vacuity of the qi and yang of the spleen and kidneys, there is inadequate energy to transform and activate the uterus and the thoroughfare and controlling vessels, also leading to the inability of the egg to be fertilized or for the fertilized egg to implant itself and grow.

2. Repletion patterns

Pathogenic factors such as cold, heat, phlegm, and dampness as well as stagnation of qi and stasis of blood have the effect of obstructing the uterus and blocking its channels. Because of this blockage, fertilization cannot occur.

There is some connection between Western medical pathology and Chinese medical pathology. For example, absence or irregularity of ovulation, a small uterus, a thin endometrium, poor quality of eggs, poor quantity of follicles, low estradiol, low progesterone and high FSH, often correspond mainly to the vacuity of kidney yin, yang, or both but also correspond to qi and blood vacuity. Uterine myomas,

Traditional Chinese Medicine	Western Medicine
Vacuity of Kidney Yin or Vacuity of Blood or Vacuity of Kidney Yang or Vacuity of Qi	No Ovulation Small Uterus Thin Endometrium Poor Quality of Eggs Poor Quantity of Follicles Low Estradiol Low Progesterone High FSH
Qi Stagnation or Blood Stasis or Phlegm Damp Obstruction	Fallopian Tube Block Uterine Fibroid Ovarian Cystitis Endometriosis Adhesions Stress
Damp Heat or Toxins or Blood Stasis	Cervical Infection Vaginal Infection Pelvic Infection Fallopian Tube Infection

Figure 4.

ovarian cystitis, adhesions, endometriosis, and blockage of fallopian tubes often correspond to the Chinese medical pattern discrimination of qi stagnation and blood stasis with phlegm dampness. Cervical infection, vaginal infection, pelvic infection and fallopian tube infection often correspond to damp heat or toxins with blood stasis.

Western medical pathologies of male reproduction

In males, there are also a number of pathological factors that may cause abnormal semen and affect fertility:

1. Testicular factors

Both testosterone and sperm are produced in the testicles. If a man has small testicles, he may produce poor quality sperm or have an insufficiency of testosterone.

A. Infection

Infections, including sexually transmitted diseases (STDs), mycoplasma, mumps, and glandular infections can all cause the sperm to become less motile.

B. Varicocele

A varicocele is an abnormally large and twisted (varicose) vein that drains blood from the testicle. It may prevent normal cooling of the testicle, thereby raising the testicular temperature. This may cause damage to the sperm.

C. Blockage of ejaculatory ducts

Some men are born with a blockage of the part of the testicle that contains sperm or ejaculatory ducts. This condition inhibits them from transferring their sperm to the female. The *vas deferens* (the tube which carries the sperm), may also be surgically blocked.

2. Sexual issues

These are general problems with sexual intercourse and technique that impair the delivery of sperm.

3. Autoimmunity

This condition occurs when immune system antibodies target sperm and weaken or disable them. A semen analysis can determine which aspect of semen function is impaired. It provides information about sperm motility, morphology, liquefaction, count, and volume.

A. Motility

Motility is the sperm's ability to move rapidly towards the egg. If this movement is impeded, the sperm will have a decreased chance of reaching the egg for fertilization. Laboratory tests* indicate that at least 50% of sperm must be able to swim to be within the normal limits. (*Test results vary, so for the purposes of this book, an average has been used.)

B. Morphology

Morphology refers to the shape and structure of the sperm. If it is abnormal, the sperm's ability to fertilize the egg may be impaired. Laboratory test results show that at least 50-70% of sperm must have a normal morphology to be considered in the normal range.

C. Liquefaction

Before ejaculation, the sperm are contained within the semen, which is thick and mucus-like. Upon ejaculation, the semen normally liquefies and becomes water-like to enable the sperm to swim towards the egg. Poor liquefaction may result from enzyme deficiencies in the seminal plasma which, in turn, reflects an abnormality of the seminal vesicles. Liquefaction should occur in less than 30 minutes to be considered normal.

D. Count

Although it only takes one sperm to fertilize an egg, a sperm count that is less than 20 million sperm per milliliter of semen is considered low. Laboratory test results require 25-250m/ml.

E. Volume

To be considered normal, the amount of semen in one ejaculation should be at least six milliliters.

Male pathology according to Chinese medicine

The following are the patterns of repletion and vacuity that affect the thoroughfare and controlling channels, which include the testicles, ejaculatory duct, the prostate, and vesicle.

1. Vacuity patterns

A. Blood & yin vacuity

A liver blood-kidney yin vacuity can impair the ability of the essence to nourish the thoroughfare and controlling channels. This may result in small testicles, low sperm count or no sperm, low volume of semen, or abnormal liquefaction.

B. Qi & yang vacuity

If there is a spleen qi-kidney yang vacuity, there is not sufficient qi to transform and activate the essence for the thoroughfare and controlling channels. This condition may cause poor motility, impotence, no ejaculation, or a testosterone deficiency.

2. Repletion patterns

A. Qi stagnation & blood stasis

In this condition, qi stagnation and blood stasis can obstruct the thoroughfare and controlling vessels leading to poor morphology, varicocele, or blockage of the ejaculatory ducts.

B. Damp heat

Replete damp heat evils can also damage the thoroughfare and controlling vessels, killing the sperm.

There is a correlation between Chinese and Western medical pathologies. What Western medicine would call sexual issues, failure to ejaculate, autoimmunity, small testicles, low testosterone levels, low semen volume, low sperm count, low quality sperm, or abnormal motility, Chinese medicine views as a vacuity of the kidneys or as a vacuity of qi and blood. Abnormal morphology, varicocele, or blockage of ejaculatory ducts correspond to the Chinese medical differentiation of qi stagnation or blood stasis. Infections are typically caused by what Chinese medicine labels damp heat pathogens.

Traditional Chinese Medicine	Western Medicine
Vacuity of Kidney Yin or Vacuity of Qi and Blood	Sexual Issues No Ejaculate Autoimmunity Small Testicles Testosterone Vacuity Low Semen Volume Low Sperm Count Low Quality Sperm Abnormal Motility
Qi Stagnation or Blood Stasis	Abnormal Morphology Varicocele Blockage of Ejaculatory Ducts
Dampness and Heat	Infection

Figure 5.

3

Procedures of *In Vitro* Fertilization

Human *in vitro* fertilization is a process in which the egg and sperm are fertilized *in vitro*, meaning outside of the body in a petri dish. (*In vitro* literally means in glass.) The fertilized embryo is then implanted into the female's uterus. IVF was first successful in the United States in 1981. Since then, it has become a widely accepted method of treatment for infertile couples.

There are various causes of infertility, many of which can successfully be treated with IVF. The indications for *in vitro* fertilization include:

Fallopian tube obstruction
Oligospermia (low sperm count)
Abnormal cervical factor
Immunologic factor—husband or wife
Unexplained infertility
Infertility after tubal surgery
Infertility after treatment for endometriosis

The following is an overview of the steps of IVF:

1. Regulation of hormones

Once pretreatment screening of a couple has taken place, the IVF specialist or team will attempt to regulate and control the hormones prior to beginning IVF. There are many different methods to performing the various steps with *in vitro* fertilization. Presently, the most common method is for female patients to take oral contraceptive pills for the first month. Recently, there have been some physicians who do not give birth control pills to women over age 40 or if they have high FSH levels. When trying to control ovulation, one common method is for the patient to take leuprolide acetate (Lupron) before or after stopping birth control pills. Another current method is to give ganerelix (Antagon) three days prior to the hCG (human chorionic gonadotropin) injection to control ovulation.

2. Stimulation of ovulation

There is a choice of basic stimulation protocols available to the patient and physician. There is no single approach to ovulation stimulation that works equally well for all patients. Physicians will be guided by the person's medical history, and perhaps also by previous responses to those agents, in determining the stimulation protocol best suited for each patient. Even when the woman has normal ovulatory function, ovulation stimulation will be employed in almost all cases in order to induce development of the maximum number of follicles containing mature oocytes. Commonly used drugs, such as menotropins (Pergonal or Repronex), follitropin beta (Follistim), and follitropin-alpha (Gonal-F), are given to stimulate the ovaries to produce more follicles and regulate the hormones. Pergonal and Repronex contain both the LH (luteinizing hormone) and FSH (follicle-stimulating hormone), while Follistim and Gonal-F contain only FSH.

3. Monitoring follicular development

During the stimulation phase, the ovarian response is usually monitored with some combination of ultrasound examinations to track follicular development and blood tests to measure hormone levels (primarily estrogen and LH). As the follicles mature, these tests may be performed daily over a 4-6 day interval.

During the final stages of follicular development and egg maturation, the patient will be given a hCG (human chorionic gonadotropin) injection. This is timed 34-36 hours prior to the egg retrieval, just before ovulation would occur, and helps to change immature eggs into mature or metaphase II eggs.

4. Oocyte retrieval

Various techniques have been used for oocyte aspiration. In the past, laparoscopy was usually employed. This is a procedure that makes small incisions, usually two or three, on the abdomen. Currently, the most common method being used is the transvaginal USG approach. Guided by ultrasound scanning, a physician inserts a long, thin needle through the vagina and into the ovary, thereby emptying the follicles. The needle is connected to a suction pump and the fluid from each accessible follicle within the ovary is aspirated.

Not all the eggs retrieved will be mature or normal in appearance. The percentage of eggs achieving fertilization depends on many factors. Some eggs that appear to be mature and normal in appearance will not become fertilized even when exposed to normal sperm. Not all eggs exposed to sperm will go on to division (cleavage). Not all eggs fertilize and even those that do may not all continue to divide beyond the four cell stage. As an example, a typical cycle may produce twelve eggs of which eight become fertilized and seven begin to divide in a satisfactory fashion. Depending on the female patient's age, 2-4 will be transferred to the uterus and two or three will be cryopreserved (frozen).

5. Laboratory component

If the follicle is mature, a visible amount of granulosa cells will accompany the aspirated fluid in which the mature ovum is found. This fluid is examined by an embryologist under a microscope in order to identify and isolate the egg complex. The oocyte is identified and graded for its maturity, placed in an incubation medium within a petri dish, and finally transferred into the incubator. Eggs are usually cultured in the incubator for 3-6 hours depending on maturity before being exposed to sperm.

For semen, various forms of preparation can be used, from a simple washing and centrifugation, to a more complicated "swim-up" procedure that separates only motile sperm to be used for insemination. To perform insemination, between 50,000-500,000 motile sperm per milliliter are needed. When sperm quality and/or numbers are low, it may be necessary to hold the egg under the microscope and inject a single sperm into the interior of the egg (a procedure known as intracytoplasmic sperm injection or ICSI).

6. Embryo growth in culture

Once the oocyte has been fertilized with the sperm, it is examined approximately 15-18 hours later for fertilization and switched from the incubation medium to a growth medium that contains twice the amount of protein. Next, the fertilized egg is returned to the incubator and kept there until the time of transfer, usually around 48-72 hours after insemination. The fertilized egg is ordinarily in the four or eight-cell stage before transfer of the embryo can take place.

7. Embryo transfer

Approximately 2-6 days after insemination, the dividing embryos selected for replacement in the uterus are loaded into a soft plastic catheter. Using a small volume of medium, the biologist loads the catheter and the physician passes it through the cervix wall into the uterine cavity. Most programs transfer 2-3 embryos in patients under age 35 undergoing their first cycle of treatment, and 3-4 in those ages 35-40 to maximize their chance of success while minimizing multiple pregnancies. Additional healthy embryos may be frozen in liquid nitrogen to be used later if implantation and pregnancy do not occur.

8. Luteal phase monitoring

After ovulation has occurred, supplemental progesterone in the form of vaginal suppositories, injections, or micronized oral tablets may be added. Ultrasonography may be employed to measure ovarian size, particularly if hyperstimulation is suspected.

Pregnancy testing is usually performed 12-14 days after egg retrieval. If the results are positive, progesterone levels will be checked and the pregnancy test repeated in order to measure the rate of rise in hCG that occurs in early pregnancy. Using vaginal ultrasonography, a fetal sac typically can be seen 25 days following egg retrieval, and by the 35th day, fetal heart motion can be observed.

4

Chinese Medical Preparation Before
In Vitro Fertilization: Females

Approximately three months prior to the IVF procedure, it is recommended that the patient receive acupuncture and herbal treatments to regulate the body's functions and make IVF more successful.
Sometimes after just these three months, the patient regains a normal
menstrual cycle and is able to become pregnant naturally.

During the three months preparation time, the main objectives of
Chinese medical therapy are to:

1. Improve the function of the ovaries

Acupuncture and Chinese medicinals help to improve ovarian function, allowing for development of better quality eggs and strong,
healthy embryos. Chinese medicine can also regulate estrogen and
progesterone levels, thereby thickening the lining of the uterus.
Research indicates increased blood flow to the uterus can help promote
follicular development and also implantation of the embryo.

Acupuncture and Chinese medicinals can help the ovaries respond better to the stimulating drugs by producing more follicles and good quality eggs. Many patients using IVF alone are only able to produce a few
follicles. Based on clinical experience, we estimate that Chinese medicine can help the ovaries *at least double* the number of follicles as well
as significantly enhance the embryo's quality and quantity.

High FSH levels indicate poor ovarian function. Chinese medicine is
able to help decrease the FSH levels by regulating the hormones and
function of the ovaries. Before treatment can begin, the practitioner
should check the FSH level in the patient's medical history. A high

number may suggest the lack of ovulation as hormones continue to increase to stimulate the ovaries to work harder. The normal range should remain below ten. Any test reading above 35 may indicate menopause.

2. Strengthen the immune system & reduce stress

Approximately half of chemical pregnancies miscarry. Therefore, one of the key treatment strategies is to strengthen the patient's immune system through acupuncture and herbs.

Many patients using IVF drugs experience side effects and high levels of stress associated with trying to get pregnant. Chinese medicine is extremely helpful in reducing stress and alleviating side effects, which helps the patient be calmer and more at ease. Relaxing the patient helps prevent the uterus from contracting, thereby improving the implantation process and preventing miscarriage.

3. Improve semen quality & quantity

Sperm maturation is a process taking between 70-90 days. It is also important for male patients to prepare for IVF during this time period. Chinese medicine can help male patients improve the quality and quantity of semen (see Chapter 5). In so doing, the health of the embryo improves, which in turn reduces the risk of miscarriage.

4. Diet & lifestyle

In Chinese medicine, diet and exercise are seen as important components in maintaining health. Dietary suggestions include a reduction in cold drinks and raw foods as well as limiting the intake of ice cream, chocolate, and coffee. I recommend cooking chicken soup with ginger, beans, and vegetables and including this in the diet to help nourish the uterus. I also suggest fish soup with ginger to improve the quantity and quality of semen. In addition, it is important to eat meals on a regular schedule.

Exercise is another beneficial lifestyle change that relieves stress and can improve the health of the body and, thereby, increase the chances of getting pregnant. Some traditional Chinese exercises include *tai ji*, *qi gong*, and meditation. Another type of recommended exercise is yoga.

Clinical protocols:

Chinese medicine is very successful in treating many gynecological disorders that accompany and contribute to infertility, such as irregular menstruation, amenorrhea, endometriosis, uterine fibroids, and heavy bleeding (metrorrhagia) due to anovulation. Along with physical complications and an imbalance of hormones, these disorders can affect a patient's ability to become pregnant. By treating the root causes of infertility, some patients may become pregnant naturally during the preparation time. For others, the chance of a successful IVF outcome is significantly increased.

The following pages discuss the formulas I have found the most clinically useful for preparing a patient for IVF. For historical perspective and as a reference tool, classical formulas for female infertility are discussed later in this chapter.

In terms of acupuncture, the points given below are recommended for preparing most female patients for IVF:

Zu San Li (St 36), *San Yin Jiao* (Sp 6), *Tai Chong* (Liv 3), *He Gu* (LI 4), *Di Ji* (Sp 8), and *Yin Tang* (M-HN-3)

Modifications:

If there is more yang vacuity, add *Ming Men* (GV 4) and *Fu Liu* (Ki 7). For more yin vacuity, add *Tai Xi* (Ki 3).

Formula rationale:

Zu San Li rectifies the digestion and supports the defensive qi (*i.e.*, the immune system). *San Yin Jiao* offers access to the liver, kidney, and spleen channels and nourishes blood. *Tai Chong* used with *He Gu* is known as the Four Bars or Gates. This combination strongly courses and rectifies the liver qi. *Di Ji* helps regulate the hormones, and *Yin Tang* is used to help relax the patient's mind and emotions. *Ming Men* and *Fu Liu* effectively invigorate kidney yang, while *Tai Xi* is the source point of the kidney channel, meaning that it strongly supplements the source qi of the kidneys.

In addition to the above points, further suggestions will be provided specific to the patient's situation.

1. Early/delayed/erratic menstruation.

Menstrual cycles may range from 21-40 days, although the average range is from 24-32 days. The formula *Ding Jing Fang* (Stabilize Menstruation Formula) can be given for all three diagnoses of early, delayed, or irregular menstruation but with modifications in timing and herbs.

Ding Jing Fang is based on Fu Qing-zhu's famous Qing dynasty formula *Ding Jing Tang* (Stabilize Menstruation Decoction). According to Fu Qing-zhu, this formula soothes the liver and resolves depression which then opens depression of the kidney qi. In *Ding Jing Fang*, blackened *Jing Jie Sui* (Herba Seu Flos Schizonepetae Tenuifoliae) is removed, since it is only used to stop heavy bleeding or prevent early menstruation. Then *Dang Shen* (Radix Codonopsitis Pilosulae), *Ba Ji Tian* (Radix Morindae Officinalis), and mix-fried *Gan Cao* (Radix Glycyrrhizae Uralanesis) are added to fortify the spleen and boost the qi, supplement the kidneys and invigorate yang. With these slight alterations, the effect of the formula is much improved to harmonize the functions of the three main viscera—spleen, liver, and kidneys—as well as supplement the qi and blood. Therefore, this formula is able to more completely treat the root of most female gynecological disorders. *Ding Jing Fang* includes:

Dang Gui (Radix Angelicae Sinensis)
Bai Shao (Radix Albus Paeoniae Lactiflorae)
Shu Di Huang (cooked Radix Rehmanniae Glutinosae)
Chai Hu (Radix Bupleuri)
Shan Yao (Radix Dioscoreae Oppositae)
Fu Ling (Sclerotium Poriae Cocos)
Tu Si Zi (Semen Cuscutae Chinensis)
mix-fried *Gan Cao* (Radix Glycyrrhizae Uralanesis)
Dang Shen (Radix Codonopsitis Pilosulae)
Ba Ji Tian (Radix Morindae Officinalis)

Formula rationale:

Within this formula, *Dang Gui* nourishes and quickens the blood. *Bai Shao* nourishes the blood, harmonizes the liver and constrains yin. *Shu Di Huang* nourishes the blood and supplements the kidneys, enriches yin and fosters essence. *Chai Hu* courses the liver and rectifies the qi. *Shan Yao* supplements both the spleen and kidney qi while engendering fluids. *Fu Ling* fortifies the spleen and quiets the spirit. *Tu Si Zi* supplements the kidneys and enriches yin, invigorates yang and boosts the essence. Mix-fried *Gan Cao* supplements the qi and harmonizes all the other ingredients in the formula. *Dang Shen* fortifies the spleen and boosts the qi, while *Ba Ji Tian* gently supplements and invigorates kidney yang and essence.

A. Early menstruation

The formula *Ding Jing Fang* is given one week before the patient's own cycle begins. For example, if the patient's cycle is usually 20 days, start *Ding Jing Fang* on the 13th day of her cycle. Other modifications can be made to push back the cycle and prevent bleeding as listed below:

Modifications:

For kidney yin vacuity and vacuity heat, add *Han Lian Cao* (Herba Ecliptae Prostratae) and *Nu Zhen Zi* (Fructus Ligustri Lucidi). This latter combination is also known as *Er Zhi Wan* (Two Ultimates Pills). For spleen qi vacuity (failing to manage the blood), add *Huang Qi* (Radix Astragali Membranacei). For blood vacuity, add *E Jiao* (Gelatinum Corii Asini). For blood heat, add *Ce Bai Ye* (Cacumen Biotae Orientalis) or *Di Yu* (Radix Sanguisorbae Officinalis).

Additional points:

Bai Hui (GV 20) to upbear and lift the clear yang so as to contain the blood. Ear: Endocrine, *Shen Men*

B. Delayed menstruation

Ding Jing Fang is taken one week before the normal cycle (consisting of 28 days) begins or on the 21st day of the cycle. For example, if the patient's cycle is usually 40 days, the formula is started on the 21st day. This formula will help bring the menses to arrive at regular 28-30 day cycles.

Modifications:

For blood stasis, add *Dan Shen* (Radix Salviae Miltiorrhizae), *Chuan*

Xiong (Radix Ligustici Wallichii), *Niu Xi* (Radix Achyranthis Bidentatae), *Mu Dan Pi* (Cortex Radicis Moutan), and *Chi Shao* (Radix Rubrus Paeoniae Lactiflorae). For qi stagnation, add *Xiang Fu* (Rhizoma Cyperi Rotundi), *Yu Jin* (Tuber Curcumae), and *Zhi Ke* (Fructus Citri Aurantii). For vacuity cold caused by yang vacuity, add *Yin Yang Huo* (Herba Epimedii) and *Rou Gui* (Cortex Cinnamomi Cassiae). For repletion cold, add *Gan Jiang* (dry Rhizoma Zingiberis Officinalis), *Xiao Hui Xiang* (Fructus Foeniculi Vulgaris), and *Gui Zhi* (Ramulus Cinnamomi Cassiae). For blood vacuity, add *Ji Xue Teng* (Radix Et Caulis Jixueteng), *Gou Qi Zi* (Fructus Lycii Chinensis), *He Shou Wu* (Radix Polygoni Multiflori), and *Huang Jing* (Rhizoma Polygonati).

Additional points:

Xue Hai (Sp 10) to quicken the blood and *Guan Yuan* (CV 4) and *Qi Hai* (CV 6) to move the qi downward and regulate menstruation

C. Erratic menstruation (*i.e.*, sometimes early, sometimes late, no fixed schedule menstruation)

Xiao Yao Fang (Rambling Formula, a.k.a. *Xiao Yao San*, Rambling Powder) should be taken for three weeks beginning right after the menstruation is over. This formula courses the liver and rectifies the qi, fortifies the spleen, supplements the qi, and both nourishes and quickens the blood, thereby regulating the menses. It consists of:

Chai Hu (Radix Bupleuri)
Dang Gui (Radix Angelicae Sinensis)
Bai Shao (Radix Albus Paeoniae Lactiflorae)
Bai Zhu (Rhizoma Atractylodis Macrocephalae)
Fu Ling (Sclerotium Poriae Cocos)
Gan Cao (Radix Glycyrrhizae Uralanesis)
Sheng Jiang (uncooked Rhizoma Zingiberis Officinalis)

Formula rationale:

Within this formula, *Chai Hu* courses the liver and rectifies the qi. *Dang Gui* nourishes and quickens the blood. *Bai Shao* nourishes the blood, harmonizes the liver, and constrains yin. *Bai Zhu* fortifies the spleen and supplements the qi. *Fu Ling* fortifies the spleen and quiets the spirit. *Gan Cao* supplements the qi as well as harmonizes all the other medicinals in the formula. *Sheng Jiang* warms and harmonizes the spleen and stomach.

Modifications:

For marked qi vacuity, add *Dang Shen* (Radix Codonopsitis Pilosulae). For concomitant kidney yin vacuity, add *Shu Di Huang* (cooked Radix Rehmanniae Glutinosae), *Shan Zhu Yu* (Fructus Corni Officinalis), and *Nu Zhen Zi* (Fructus Ligustri Lucidi). For concomitant kidney yang vacuity, add *Ba Ji Tian* (Radix Morindae Officinalis), *Yin Yang Huo* (Herba Epimedii), and *Rou Cong Rong* (Herba Cistanchis Deserticolae). For kidney yin and yang vacuity, add *Tu Si Zi* (Semen Cuscutae Chinensis). For blood vacuity, add *Gou Qi Zi* (Fructus Lycii Chinensis), *He Shou Wu* (Radix Polygoni Multiflori), and *Huang Jing* (Rhizoma Polygonati). For qi stagnation, add *Xiang Fu* (Rhizoma Cyperi Rotundi), *Yu Jin* (Tuber Curcumae), and/or *Zhi Ke* (Fructus Citri Aurantii), and for blood stasis, add *Dan Shen* (Radix Salviae Miltiorrhizae) and *Ji Xue Teng* (Radix Et Caulis Jixueteng).

Additional points:

One may substitute *Qu Quan* (Liv 8) for *Tai Chong* (Liv 3) to course the liver and move the qi more strongly. If performing acupuncture on the back, use *Pi Shu* (Bl 20), *Shen Shu* (Bl 23), and *Da Chang Shu* (Bl 25).

2. Amenorrhea

Amenorrhea is defined as the absence of menstruation. Primary amenorrhea refers to menstruation that never starts. Secondary amenorrhea refers to menstruation that ceases to occur for more than three consecutive months after menarche has occurred. In Chinese medicine, amenorrhea can be caused by such disease mechanisms as kidney yin, yang, or essence vacuity, qi and blood vacuity, binding depression of the liver qi with blood stasis, and phlegm obstruction. The treatment protocol, based on clinical experience, is divided into two steps.

Step 1 is to quicken and nourish the blood and course the qi for one week, presumably days 21-28 if that is ascertainable. For these purposes, we can use the formula *Jing Qian Fang* (Menstruation-smoothing Formula):

Dang Gui (Radix Angelicae Sinensis)
Bai Shao (Radix Albus Paeoniae Lactiflorae)
Shu Di Huang (cooked Radix Rehmanniae Glutinosae)
Gou Qi Zi (Fructus Lycii Chinensis)
Chuan Xiong (Radix Ligustici Wallichii)
Niu Xi (Radix Achyranthis Bidentatae)
Dan Shen (Radix Salviae Miltiorrhizae)
Xiang Fu (Rhizoma Cyperi Rotundi)

Formula rationale:

Within this formula, *Dang Gui* nourishes and quickens the blood. *Bai Shao* nourishes the blood, harmonizes the liver, and constrains yin. *Shu Di Huang* nourishes the blood and enriches yin, supplements the kidneys and fosters the essence. *Gou Qi Zi* nourishes liver yin and blood. *Chuan Xiong* moves the qi and quickens the blood. *Niu Xi* and *Dan Shen* both quicken the blood and transform stasis. *Xiang Fu* courses the liver, rectifies the qi, and regulates menstruation.

Modifications:

For marked qi vacuity, add *Dang Shen* (Radix Codonopsitis Pilosulae). For yang vacuity, add *Ba Ji Tian* (Radix Morindae Officinalis) and *Yin Yang Huo* (Herba Epimedii). For bood vacuity, add *Ji Xue Teng* (Radix Et Caulis Jixueteng), *Huang Jing* (Rhizoma Polygonati), and *He Shou Wu* (Radix Polygoni Multiflori). For qi stagnation, add *Zhi Ke* (Fructus Citri Aurantii) and *Yu Jin* (Tuber Curcumae). For blood stasis, add *Wang Bu Liu Xing* (Semen Vaccariae Segetalis), *Mu Dan Pi* (Cortex Radicis Moutan), and *Chi Shao* (Radix Rubrus Paeoniae Lactiflorae). For cold in the abdomen (a.k.a. uterine cold), add *Xiao Hui Xiang* (Fructus Foeniculi Vulgaris) and *Rou Gui* (Cortex Cinnamomi Cassiae) or *Gui Zhi* (Ramulus Cinnamomi Cassiae).

Additional points:

Zhong Ji (CV 3), *Guan Yuan* (CV 4), and/or *Qi Hai* (CV 6) to course the qi and move it downward and *Xue Hai* (Sp 10) to quicken the blood. If there is uterine cold, one can add moxa to the controlling vessel points above.

Step 2 is to supplement the kidneys and nourish the blood, fortify the spleen and course the liver for three weeks using the formula *Ding Jing Fang* for days 1-20 of the cycle. This formula helps build the uterine lining so that menstruation can occur.

Dang Gui (Radix Angelicae Sinensis)
Bai Shao (Radix Albus Paeoniae Lactiflorae)
Shu Di Huang (cooked Radix Rehmanniae Glutinosae)
Chai Hu (Radix Bupleuri)
Shan Yao (Radix Dioscoreae Oppositae)
Fu Ling (Sclerotium Poriae Cocos)
Tu Si Zi (Semen Cuscutae Chinensis)
mix-fried *Gan Cao* (Radix Glycyrrhizae Uralanesis)
Dang Shen (Radix Codonopsitis Pilosulae)
Ba Ji Tian (Radix Morindae Officinalis)

Modifications:

For qi vacuity, add *Huang Qi* (Radix Astragali Membranacei). For kidney yin vacuity, add *Shan Zhu Yu* (Fructus Corni Officinalis), *Nu Zhen Zi* (Fructus Ligustri Lucidi), and *Sang Shen Zi* (Fructus Mori Albi). For kidney yang vacuity, add *Rou Cong Rong* (Herba Cistanchis Deserticolae), *Yin Yang Huo* (Herba Epimedii), and *Suo Yang* (Herba Cynomorii Songarici). For kidney yin and yang vacuity, add *Zi He Che* (Placenta Hominis) and *Sha Yuan Zi* (Semen Astragali Complanati). For blood vacuity, add *Huang Jing* (Rhizoma Polygonati), *He Shou Wu* (Radix Polygoni Multiflori), *Ji Xue Teng* (Radix Et Caulis Jixueteng), and *Gou Qi Zi* (Fructus Lycii Chinensis). For qi stagnation, add *Xiang Fu* (Rhizoma Cyperi Rotundi), *Zhi Ke* (Fructus Citri Aurantii), and *Yu Jin* (Tuber Curcumae). For fluid dryness, add *Mai Men Dong* (Tuber Ophiopogonis Japonici), *Sheng Di Huang* (uncooked Radix Rehmanniae Glutinosae), and *Xuan Shen* (Radix Scrophulariae Ningpoensis). For insomnia, add *Suan Zao Ren* (Semen Zizyphi Spinosae), *Wu Wei Zi* (Fructus Schisandrae Chinensis), and *Long Yan Rou* (Arillus Euphoriae Longanae) or *Bai Zi Ren* (Semen Biotae Orientalis). For abdominal distention, add *Chen Pi* (Pericarpium Citri Reticulatae) or *Sha Ren* (Fructus Amomi).

This idea is similar to that of oral contraceptive pills but is different in that it is not hormone replacement but, rather, these formulas help to regulate the endocrine system and stimulate the ovaries to bring about normal ovulation and regular menstrual cycles.

Additional points:

Bai Hui (GV 20) to stimulate pituitary gland. If back treatment: *Xin Shu* (Bl 15), *Ge Shu* (Bl 17), *Gan Shu* (Bl 18), *Pi Shu* (Bl 20), *Shen Shu* (Bl 23), *Da Chang Shu* (Bl 25). Ear: *Shen Men*, Kidney, Endocrine, Uterus, and halfway between Spleen and Liver

3. Endometriosis

Endometriosis is a disease in which patches of endometrial tissue, which is normally found only in the uterine lining (endometrium), grow outside the uterus. Because the misplaced endometrial tissue responds to the same hormones as the uterus, these endometrial implants can grow and can cause dysmenorrhea. The most common clinical symptoms of endometriosis are pain before and during menstruation (usually worse than "normal" menstrual cramps), pain during or after sexual intercourse (dyspareunia), infertility, and heavy or irregular menstrual bleeding. Other symptoms may include fatigue, painful bowel movements with the menstruation, lower back pain with menstruation, diarrhea and/or constipation, and other perimenstrual intestinal upset. Some women with endometriosis have no symptoms. Infertility affects about 30-40% of women with endometriosis and is a common result with progression of the disease.

Endometriosis in the ovaries is treated as if there are tumors. The blood that builds up monthly as in the endometrium lining of the uterus cannot come out of the affected ovary. The ovary then becomes cystic. If surgery is elected and the ovary is taken out, it resembles chocolate, due to its dark color and internal texture. Therefore, such endometrial cysts are also sometimes referred to as chocolate cysts. If the affected ovary is low in function, the eggs are of poor quality. Or, it may not be able to produce any eggs at all.

Endometriosis may also cause the fallopian tubes to stick together and become obstructed. However, there is a high risk of damage to the tubes if surgery is done to open them. One option for those who choose not to risk surgery is acupuncture and Chinese herbs. Using the treatment principles of quickening the blood and moving the qi, disinhibiting dampness and promoting urination (to drain liquid from the cyst), endometriosis has a high potential to be absorbed into the surrounding tissues, thus reducing or resolving the inflammation that is causing pain and infertility.

The main Chinese medical pattern discrimination for endometriosis is blood stasis. Therefore, during the whole month, the treatment principles should be to quicken the blood and dispel stasis. Yet, the use of too many blood-quickening medicinals can adversely affect the hormone levels. So it is important after the menses to slightly supplement the kidneys, nourish the blood, and fortify the spleen while still moving the qi and quickening the blood. For severe dysmenorrhea, more blood-quickening medicinals can be added just before the onset of menstruation.

Huo Jing Zhong Zi Fang (Quicken the Essence & Plant the Seed Formula) should be used for three weeks after menstruation to circulate the qi and blood, smooth the flow of the liver qi, and benefit the spleen. It includes:

Dang Gui (Radix Angelicae Sinensis)
Chai Hu (Radix Bupleuri)
Dan Shen (Radix Salviae Miltiorrhizae)
Bai Shao (Radix Albus Paeoniae Lactiflorae)
Fu Ling (Sclerotium Poriae Cocos)
Bai Zhu (Rhizoma Atractylodis Macrocephalae)
Zhi Ke (Fructus Citri Aurantii)
Gan Cao (Radix Glycyrrhizae Uralanesis)

Formula rationale:

Within this formula, *Dang Gui* helps to nourish and quicken the blood. *Chai Hu* enters the liver channel where it courses the liver and rectifies the qi. *Dan Shen* moves the blood and quiets the spirit. *Bai Shao* nourishes and emolliates the liver, and constrains yin. *Fu Ling* fortifies the spleen and quiets the spirit, while *Bai Zhu* helps fortify the spleen and supplement the qi. *Zhi Ke* rectifies the qi, and *Gan Cao* harmonizes all the other ingredients in the formula.

31

Modifications:

For spleen vacuity, add *Dang Shen* (Radix Codonopsitis Pilosulae) and/or *Huang Qi* (Radix Astragali Membranacei). For kidney vacuity, add *Nu Zhen Zi* (Fructus Ligustri Lucidi), *Sang Ji Sheng* (Ramulus Sangjisheng), and *Xu Duan* (Radix Dipsaci Asperi). For qi stagnation, add *Yu Jin* (Tuber Curcumae) and *Xiang Fu* (Rhizoma Cyperi Rotundi). For blood stasis, add *Chi Shao* (Radix Rubrus Paeoniae Lactiflorae), *Mu Dan Pi* (Cortex Radicis Moutan), and *San Qi* (Radix Notoginseng). For blood vacuity, add *Gou Qi Zi* (Fructus Lycii Chinensis) and *Ji Xue Teng* (Radix Et Caulis Jixueteng).

Additional points:

Xue Hai (Sp 10) and *Qu Quan* (Liv 8) to help quicken the blood and *Zi Gong Xue* (M-CA-18) to improve ovarian circulation.

Xiao Zheng Fang (Disperse Concretions Formula) should then be used for one week immediately before the onset of menstruation and during the menstrual period itself (approximately days 25 through the 4th or 5th day of the cycle):

Ji Xue Teng (Radix Et Caulis Jixueteng)
San Leng (Rhizoma Sparganii Stoloniferi*)*
E Zhu (Rhizoma Curcumae Ezhu)
Mu Dan Pi (Cortex Radicis Moutan)
Dan Shen (Radix Salviae Miltiorrhizae)
Chi Shao (Radix Rubrus Paeoniae Lactiflorae)
Tao Ren (Semen Pruni Persicae)
Zhi Ke (Fructus Citri Aurantii)
Fu Ling (Sclerotium Poriae Cocos)
Bai Zhu (Rhizoma Atractylodis Macrocephalae)

Formula rationale:

Within this formula, *Ji Xue Teng* nourishes and quickens the blood. *San Leng* forcefully breaks the blood and moves the qi. *E Zhu* also quickens the blood and breaks stasis while rectifying the qi. *Mu Dan Pi* quickens the blood. *Dan Shen* and *Chi Shao* quicken the blood and dispel stasis. *Tao Ren* quickens the blood and moistens the intestines. *Zhi Ke* courses the liver, moves the qi, and resolves depression. *Fu Ling* disinhibits dampness, fortifies the spleen, and quiets the spirit, and *Bai Zhu* fortifies the spleen and supplements the qi.

Modifications:

For qi stagnation, add *Xiang Fu* (Rhizoma Cyperi Rotundi) and *Yu Jin* (Tuber Curcumae). For blood stasis, add *Wang Bu Liu Xing* (Semen Vaccariae Segetalis) and *Hong Hua* (Flos Carthami Tinctorii). To promote urination, add *Yi Yi Ren* (Semen Coicis Lachryma-jobi), *Mu Tong* (Caulis Akebiae), *Che Qian Zi* (Semen Plantaginis), and *Ze Xie* (Rhizoma Alismatis Orientalis). To dry dampness, add *Ban Xia* (Rhizoma Pinelliae Ternatae), *Chen Pi* (Pericarpium Citri Reticulatae), and *Cang Zhu* (Rhizoma Atractylodis). For severe menstrual pain, add *Yan Hu Suo* (Rhizoma Corydalis Yanhusuo), *Mo Yao* (Resina Myrrhae), and *Ru Xiang* (Resina Olibani). For heavy bleeding, add *Pu Huang* (Pollen Typhae), *Wu Ling Zhi* (Excrementum Trogopteri Seu Pteromi), *Yi Mu Cao* (Herba Leonuri Heterophylli), and *San Qi* (Radix Notoginseng). For cold in the abdomen, add *Xiao Hui Xiang* (Fructus Foeniculi Vulgaris) and *Rou Gui* (Cortex Cinnamomi Cassiae) or *Gui Zhi* (Ramulus Cinnamomi Cassiae).

Additional points:

Zhong Ji (CV 3) or *Guan Yuan* (CV 4) to help free the flow of the menses and reduce dysmenorrhea and *Xue Hai* (Sp 10) to help quicken the blood.

4. Uterine myomas

Uterine myomas or fibroids are nodules of smooth muscle cells and fibrous connective tissue that develop within the wall of the uterus. Most of the time uterine myomas are not dangerous. The masses are benign tumors not associated with an increased risk of uterine cancer and almost never develop into cancer. The factors that initiate uterine myoma growth are unknown, but myomas do seem to be affected by estrogen levels, often growing larger during pregnancy and shrinking after menopause. Uterine myomas may or may not cause symptoms. These may include heavy or prolonged menstrual bleeding, pain or heaviness in the pelvic area during or between menstrual periods, swelling of the abdomen, a need to urinate more frequently, and infertility caused by blockage of the fallopian tubes or distortion of the uterine cavity.

In Chinese medicine, *zheng jia* (literally, concretions and conglomerations) primarily refer to uterine masses. The two manifestations included in the diagnosis are uterine fibroids and ovarian cysts. Concretions refers to a "true" mass which is hard, fixed in location, and accompanied by localized pain. The disease mechanism behind this disorder is primarily blood stasis. Conglomeration refers to a "false" mass that is movable, comes and goes, has an indistinct form, and cannot be palpated. Conglomerations are mostly due to qi stagnation. The treatment of fibroids and cysts differs slightly based upon individual etiology.

The treatment principles for uterine fibroids and ovarian cysts in Chinese medicine are to break stagnation and transform stasis. The formula used to treat uterine fibroids is *Xiao Zheng Fang* (Disperse Concretions Formula):

Ji Xue Teng (Radix Et Caulis Jixueteng)
San Leng (Rhizoma Sparganii Stoloniferi)
E Zhu (Rhizoma Curcumae Ezhu)
Mu Dan Pi (Cortex Radicis Moutan)
Dan Shen (Radix Salviae Miltiorrhizae)
Chi Shao (Radix Rubrus Paeoniae Lactiflorae)
Tao Ren (Semen Pruni Persicae)
Zhi Ke (Fructus Citri Aurantii)
Fu Ling (Sclerotium Poriae Cocos)
Bai Zhu (Rhizoma Atractylodis Macrocephalae)

Modifications:

For qi stagnation, add *Chai Hu* (Radix Bupleuri), *Xiang Fu* (Rhizoma Cyperi Rotundi), *Qing Pi* (Pericarpium Citri Reticulatae Viride), and/or *Li Zhi He* (Semen Litchi Chinensis). For blood stasis, add *Wang Bu Liu Xing* (Semen Vaccariae Segetalis), *Hong Hua* (Flos Carthami Tinctorii), *Chuan Xiong* (Radix Ligustici Wallichii), and *Yan Hu Suo* (Rhizoma Corydalis Yanhusuo). For phlegm, add *Cang Zhu* (Rhizoma Atractylodis), *Ban Xia* (Rhizoma Pinelliae Ternatae), *Chen Pi* (Pericarpium Citri Reticulatae), *Chuan Bei Mu* (Bulbus Fritillariae Cirrhosae), *Hai Zao* (Herba Sargassii), and *Kun Bu* (Thallus Algae). For dampness, add *Yi Yi Ren* (Semen Coicis Lachryma-jobi), *Mu Tong* (Caulis Akebiae), *Ze Xie* (Rhizoma Alismatis Orientalis), *Zhu Ling* (Sclerotium Polypori Umbellati), *Che Qian Zi* (Semen Plantaginis), and

Qu Mai (Herba Dianthi). For menorrhagia, add *Pu Huang* (Pollen Typhae), *Wu Ling Zhi* (Excrementum Trogopteri Seu Pteromi), *San Qi* (Radix Notoginseng), *Yi Mu Cao* (Herba Leonuri Heterophylli), *Xue Yu Tan* (Crinis Carbonisatus), and carbonized *Shan Zha* (Fructus Crataegi).

Note: Do not use kidney channel points since these will stimulate the hormones and this can aggravate accumulation of fibroids.

Additional points:

Xue Hai (Sp 10) to quicken the blood and *Qu Quan* to move the qi. If there are fluid-filled cysts, use *Yin Ling Quan* to drain dampness, *Feng Long* (St 40) to transform phlegm, and *Wai Guan* (TB 5) to assist fluid circulation.

5. Heavy uterine bleeding due to anovulation

Heavy uterine bleeding may occur during menstruation (menorrhagia) or in between menstrual periods (metrorrhagia). In many cases, heavy uterine bleeding can be caused by a lack of ovulation, resulting in infertility. With anovulation, the treatment principles are to regulate the hormone levels to encourage ovulation of the ovaries, thereby normalizing menstrual bleeding. The four main Chinese medical patterns describing heavy uterine bleeding are spleen qi vacuity, kidney vacuity, blood heat, and blood stasis. Spleen qi vacuity is unable to hold the blood within its vessels thus causing heavy uterine bleeding. In kidney vacuity, heavy bleeding is caused by the kidneys not being able to secure the essence which helps form the blood. Heat in the blood forces it to move frenetically outside of the vessels, thus also bringing upon heavy uterine bleeding. Lastly, static blood prevents the blood vessels from constricting, therefore causing continuous, heavy bleeding.

The basic formula to treat heavy uterine bleeding is *Gong Xue Fang* (Uterine Bleeding Formula) which consists of:

Dang Shen (Radix Codonopsitis Pilosulae)
Bai Zhu (Rhizoma Atractylodis Macrocephalae)
Xu Duan (Radix Dipsaci Asperi)
Shan Zhu Yu (Fructus Corni Officinalis)

Formula rationale:

Within this formula, *Dang Shen* supplements the qi thereby managing or containing the blood within its channels. *Bai Zhu* fortifies the spleen to help manage the blood. *Xu Duan* supplements and invigorates kidney yang and *Shan Zhu Yu* supplements and enriches kidney yin. Together they control the essence in order to store the blood.

Modifications:

For qi vacuity, add *Huang Qi* (Radix Astragali Membranacei) and *Ren Shen* (Radix Panacis Ginseng). For spleen vacuity, add *Shan Yao* (Radix Dioscoreae Oppositae). For kidney yin vacuity, add *Nu Zhen Zi* (Fructus Ligustri Lucidi) and *Han Lian Cao* (Herba Ecliptae Prostratae). For kidney yang vacuity, add *Lu Jiao* (Cornu Cervi) and *Bu Gu Zhi* (Fructus Psoraleae Corylifoliae). For replete heat, add *Huang Qin* (Radix Scutellariae Baicalensis). For vacuity heat, add *Sheng Di Huang* (uncooked Radix Rehmanniae Glutinosae). For blood stasis, add *Yi Mu Cao* (Herba Leonuri Heterophylli) and *San Qi* (Radix Notoginseng). For anxiety, add uncooked *Mu Li* (Concha Ostreae) and calcined *Long Gu* (Os Draconis). For coldness caused by kidney yang vacuity, add *Ai Ye* (Folium Artemisiae Argyii) and blackened *Jing Jie Sui* (Herba Seu Flos Schizonepetae Tenuifoliae).

Additional points:

Needle and moxibustion *Bai Hui* (GV 20), *Da Dun* (Liv 1), *Yin Bai* (Sp 1), *Zu San Li* (St 36), *Qi Hai* (CV 6), and *Shen Que* (CV 8, moxa only)

Hemostatic or stop-bleeding medicinals may be added to treat the symptom of heavy bleeding according to each individual's pathology. For instance:

Blood heat: Add *Di Yu* (Radix Sanguisorbae Officinalis) and *Ce Bai Ye* (Cacumen Biotae Orientalis)

Blood stasis: Add *Pu Huang* (Pollen Typhae), *Wu Ling Zhi* (Excrementum Trogopteri Seu Pteromi), *Xue Yu Tan* (Crinis Carbonisatus), and carbonized *Shan Zha* (Fructus Crataegi)

Blood vacuity: Add *E Jiao* (Gelatinum Corii Asini)

Once the bleeding has stopped, it is necessary to use *Ding Jing Fang* to produce normal ovulatory cycles and prevent heavy bleeding from reoccurring. *Ding Jing Fang* includes:

Dang Gui (Radix Angelicae Sinensis)
Bai Shao (Radix Albus Paeoniae Lactiflorae)
Shu Di Huang (cooked Radix Rehmanniae Glutinosae)
Chai Hu (Radix Bupleuri)
Shan Yao (Radix Dioscoreae Oppositae)
Fu Ling (Sclerotium Poriae Cocos)
Tu Si Zi (Semen Cuscutae Chinensis)
mix-fried *Gan Cao* (Radix Glycyrrhizae Uralanesis)
Dang Shen (Radix Codonopsitis Pilosulae)
Ba Ji Tian (Radix Morindae Officinalis)

Modifications:

If there is no ovulation, add *Yin Yang Huo* (Herba Epimedii). If anovulation is due to polycystic ovary syndrome, add *Zhi Ke* (Fructus Citri Aurantii) and *Dan Shen* (Radix Salviae Miltiorrhizae) *only during ovulation*. These are added to move the qi and quicken the blood to help push the egg out of the ovary. For blood vacuity, add *He Shou Wu* (Radix Polygoni Multiflori), *Gou Qi Zi* (Fructus Lycii Chinensis), and *Huang Jing* (Rhizoma Polygonati). For poor digestion resulting in abdominal distention and bloating after meals, add *Chen Pi* (Pericarpium Citri Reticulatae) and *Sha Ren* (Fructus Amomi). For poor appetite due to concomitant food stagnation, add *Mai Ya* (Fructus Germinatus Hordei Vulgaris), *Gu Ya* (Fructus Germinatus Oryzae Sativae), and *Shan Zha* (Fructus Crataegi). For loose stools, add *Shen Qu* (Massa Medica Fermentata) and *Mu Xiang* (Radix Aucklandiae Lappae). For insomnia, add *Long Yan Rou* (Arillus Euphoriae Longanae), *Suan Zao Ren* (Semen Zizyphi Spinosae), *Bai Zi Ren* (Semen Biotae Orientalis), and *Wu Wei Zi* (Fructus Schisandrae Chinensis). For anxiety, add *Mu Li* (Concha Ostreae) and *Long Gu* (Os Draconis). For heart palpitations, add *Mai Men Dong* (Tuber Ophiopogonis Japonici) and *Dan Shen* (Radix Salviae Miltiorrhizae).

Additional points:

Bai Hui (GV 20) to help regulate the pituitary gland. Ear: Kidney, *Shen*

Men, and halfway between the Spleen and Liver. If back treatment: *Xin Shu* (Bl 15), *Ge Shu* (Bl 17), *Gan Shu* (Bl 18), *Pi Shu* (Bl 20), *Shen Shu* (Bl 23), and *Da Chang Shu* (Bl 25).

Standard Formulas

The following is a repertoire of standard Chinese medicinal formulas for regulating menstruation and treating female infertility. All of these formulas originated in the premodern literature and have been in use in China for hundreds if not thousands of years. Depending on individual situations, practitioners may choose to use one or more of these formulas in order to regulate menstruation and promote fertility instead of the formulas suggested above. While the formulas below are given in their textbook, standard form, in real life they are typically modified with additions and subtractions depending on the particular needs and presentation of each patient.

1. Early menstruation

Early menstruation refers to menstruation which consistently occurs before day 24. As the ovaries age, it is common for women to develop early menstruation due to a luteal phase defect. Traditional Chinese practice focuses on four disease mechanisms associated with early menstruation: replete heat, vacuity heat, depressive heat, and qi vacuity.

A. Replete heat

The signs and symptoms specific to replete heat are menses with a heavy, thick flow and dark red or purple-red blood. Additional symptoms may include irritability, chest oppression, abdominal distention, a red facial complexion, dry mouth, yellow urine, constipation, a red tongue with yellow fur, and a slippery, rapid pulse. The treatment principles are to clear heat and cool the blood to prevent further damage to the yin and blood. The standard formula for this condition is *Qing Jing Tang* (Clear the Menses Decoction) which is good for both replete heat and vacuity heat patterns of early menstruation:

Shu Di Huang (cooked Radix Rehmanniae Glutinosae)
Di Gu Pi (Cortex Radicis Lycii Chinensis)
Mu Dan Pi (Cortex Radicis Moutan)

Bai Shao (Radix Albus Paeoniae Lactiflorae)
Qing Hao (Herba Artemisiae Annuae)
Huang Bai (Cortex Phellodendri)
Fu Ling (Sclerotium Poriae Cocos)

Formula rationale:

Within this formula, *Shu Di Huang* supplements the kidneys and enriches yin. *Di Gu Pi* also nourishes yin. *Mu Dan Pi* clears heat and nourishes yin. *Bai Shao* nourishes liver blood and constrains yin. *Qing Hao* clears heat and cools the blood. *Huang Bai* clears heat from the lower burner, and *Fu Ling* fortifies the spleen and quiets the spirit.

B. Vacuity heat

When vacuity heat is responsible for early menstruation, the symptoms it presents are thick, scanty, bright red blood. The treatment principles for this pattern of early menstruation are to nourish yin and clear vacuity heat. *Liang Di Tang* (Dual Rehmannia Decoction) is the standard formula commonly used:

Sheng Di Huang (uncooked Radix Rehmanniae Glutinosae)
Di Gu Pi (Cortex Radicis Lycii Chinensis)
Xuan Shen (Radix Scrophulariae Ningpoensis)
Bai Shao (Radix Albus Paeoniae Lactiflorae)
Mai Men Dong (Tuber Ophiopogonis Japonici)

Formula rationale:

Within this formula, *Sheng Di Huang* nourishes yin and cools the blood. *Di Gu Pi* clears vacuity heat and nourishes yin. *Xuan Shen* likewise supplements and nourishes kidney yin. *Bai Shao* emolliates the liver and constrains yin. *Mai Men Dong* also nourishes yin. One can modify this formula with the addition of *E Jiao* (Gelatinum Corii Asini) to further nourish yin and blood and stop bleeding to help prevent the menses from occurring early.

C. Depressive heat

Symptoms of this pattern include menses with a heavy or light flow which contains clots and purple-red colored blood. The patient may also experience irritability, dry mouth, heart palpitations, and lower abdominal pain. The treatment principles for this pattern are to course the liver and clear heat, fortify the spleen and nourish the blood. *Jia Wei Xiao Yao San* (Added Flavors Rambling Powder, a.k.a. *Dan Zhi Xiao Yao San,* Moutan & Gardenia Rambling Powder) includes:

Chai Hu (Radix Bupleuri)
Dang Gui (Radix Angelicae Sinensis)
Bai Shao (Radix Albus Paeoniae Lactiflorae)
Bai Zhu (Rhizoma Atractylodis Macrocephalae)
Fu Ling (Sclerotium Poriae Cocos)
Gan Cao (Radix Glycyrrhizae Uralanesis)
Sheng Jiang (uncooked Rhizoma Zingiberis Officinalis)
Bo He (Herba Menthae Haplocalycis)
Mu Dan Pi (Cortex Radicis Moutan)
Zhi Zi (Fructus Gardeniae Jasminoidis)

Formula rationale:

Within this formula, *Chai Hu* courses the liver and resolves depression. *Dang Gui* nourishes and quickens the blood. *Bai Shao* nourishes the blood, emolliates the liver, and constrains yin. *Fu Ling* fortifies the spleen and quiets the spirit. *Gan Cao* supplements the qi and harmonizes the other ingredients in the formula. *Sheng Jiang* rectifies and warms the spleen and stomach. *Bo He* courses the liver and rectifies the qi, resolves depression and clears heat. *Mu Dan Pi* clears heat, cools the blood, and promotes blood circulation. *Zhi Zi* clears heat, cools the blood, and stops bleeding.

D. Qi vacuity

The signs and symptoms characteristic of qi vacuity early menstruation are either a heavy flow of blood because the qi cannot manage the blood or a light flow due to the spleen's insufficient engenderment of the blood. The quality of blood may be fine and light or clear in color. The tongue may be pale with thin, white, possibly dry or wet fur (depending on the predominance of blood or qi vacuity). It is also possible for the tongue to be fat and enlarged with teeth-marks on its edges due to marked qi vacuity. The pulse is fine and forceless and may be bound. Additional signs may include lassitude of the spirit, fatigue, lack of strength in the four limbs, fright palpitations, shortness of breath, and constipation from the lack of qi and blood. The treatment principles for this pattern of early menstruation are to supplement the qi and blood with the classic formula *Gui Pi Tang* (Restore the Spleen Decoction):

Ren Shen (Radix Panacis Ginseng)
Bai Zhu (Rhizoma Atractylodis Macrocephalae)
Gan Cao (Radix Glycyrrhizae Uralanesis)
Huang Qi (Radix Astragali Membranacei)
Da Zao (Fructus Zizyphi Jujubae)
Dang Gui (Radix Angelicae Sinensis)
Long Yan Rou (Arillus Euphoriae Longanae)
Suan Zao Ren (Semen Zizyphi Spinosae)
Yuan Zhi (Radix Polygalae Tenuifoliae)
Fu Shen (Sclerotium Pararadicis Poriae Cocos)
Mu Xiang (Radix Aucklandiae Lappae)

Formula rationale:

Within this formula, *Ren Shen* strongly supplements qi, quiets the spirit, and generates fluids. *Bai Zhu* fortifies the spleen and supplements the qi. *Fu Shen* fortifies the spleen and quiets the spirit. *Gan Cao* supplements and boosts the spleen qi as well as harmonizes all the other ingredients in the formula. *Huang Qi* supplements the qi and blood. *Da Zao* nourishes the spleen and stomach, nourishes the blood, and quiets the spirit. *Dang Gui* nourishes and quickens the blood. *Long Yan Rou* supplements and fortifies the heart and spleen, nourishes the blood and quiets the spirit. *Suan Zao Ren* nourishes heart yin and liver blood and quiets the spirit. *Yuan Zhi* also quiets the spirit and rectifies the qi, while *Mu Xiang* harmonizes the liver and spleen and rectifies the qi.

2. Delayed menstruation

Menstruation is defined as late when the menstrual cycle is longer than 28-33 days for three consecutive months or more. The cycle may be up to 40-50 days long. There are four Chinese medical patterns associated with delayed menstruation. They include replete cold, vacuity cold, blood vacuity, and qi stagnation.

A. Replete cold

The patient may have dark-colored blood, lower abdominal pain and/or coldness, pain relieved by warmth, and normal tongue color with white fur (or coating). The flow of blood is not heavy. The traditional formula for this condition is *Wen Jing Tang* (Warm the Menses Decoction). The medicinals in this formula warm and free the flow of the blood vessels by dispersing cold, supplementing the qi, and nourishing the blood. This helps to stabilize the root of the disorder and moderately dispel stasis so that new blood may be produced, thereby relieving the problem of delayed menstruation. *Wen Jing Tang* consists of:

Ren Shen (Radix Panacis Ginseng)
Dang Gui (Radix Angelicae Sinensis)
Chuan Xiong (Radix Ligustici Wallichii)
Bai Shao (Radix Albus Paeoniae Lactiflorae)
Niu Xi (Radix Achyranthis Bidentatae)
E Zhu (Rhizoma Curcumae Ezhu)
Rou Gui (Cortex Cinnamomi Cassiae)
Mu Dan Pi (Cortex Radicis Moutan)
Gan Cao (Radix Glycyrrhizae Uralanesis)

Formula rationale:

Within this formula, *Ren Shen* strongly supplements the qi, quiets the spirit, and engenders fluids. *Dang Gui* nourishes and quickens the blood. *Chuan Xiong* moves the qi and quickens the blood. *Bai Shao* nourishes the blood and regulates menstruation, and supplements the liver and enriches yin. *Niu Xi* promotes blood circulation and moves the blood downward. *E Zhu* moves the blood, breaks stasis, and rectifies the qi. *Rou Gui* warms the channels and promotes menstruation. *Mu Dan Pi* clears heat, cools the blood, and promotes the circulation of blood. *Gan Cao* harmonizes all the other ingredients in the formula.

B. Vacuity cold

The menses are light in color and thin or clear in quality. The flow of blood is not heavy. The patient may also experience mild abdominal pain which is relieved by warmth and/or pressure. An additional sign may include a pale, swollen tongue. The treatment principles for this pattern of delayed menstruation are to supplement the blood and warm the channels with the standard formula *Da Ying Jian* (Greatly Responding Decoction):

Dang Gui (Radix Angelicae Sinensis)
Shu Di Huang (cooked Radix Rehmanniae Glutinosae)
Gou Qi Zi (Fructus Lycii Chinensis)
Du Zhong (Cortex Eucommiae Ulmoidis)
Niu Xi (Radix Achyranthis Bidentatae)
Rou Gui (Cortex Cinnamomi Cassiae)
mix-fried *Gan Cao* (Radix Glycyrrhizae Uralanesis)

Formula rationale:

Within this formula, *Dang Gui* nourishes and quickens the blood. *Shu Di Huang* nourishes the blood and enriches yin, supplements the kidneys and fosters the essence. *Gou Qi Zi* nourishes and enriches both liver blood and kidney yin. *Du Zhong* supplements and invigorates kidney yang. *Niu Xi* quickens the blood and dispels stasis. *Rou Gui* warms the channels and promotes menstruation, while mix-fried *Gan Cao* supplements the qi and harmonizes all the other ingredients in the formula.

C. Blood vacuity

The signs and symptoms of this pattern of delayed menstruation include light-colored blood, thin and clear quality of blood, and a scanty flow. Additional ailments may include weight loss, dry skin, a dry mouth, shortness of breath on exertion, fatigue, and dizziness. The treatment principles for this pattern are to boost the qi and supplement the blood, nourish the heart and calm the spirit with the famous formula *Ren Shen Yang Ying Tang* (Ginseng Nourish the Constructive Decoction):

Bai Shao (Radix Albus Paeoniae Lactiflorae)
Chuan Xiong (Radix Ligustici Wallichii)
Dang Gui (Radix Angelicae Sinensis)
Shu Di Huang (cooked Radix Rehmanniae Glutinosae)
Ren Shen (Radix Panacis Ginseng)
Bai Zhu (Rhizoma Atractylodis Macrocephalae)

Fu Ling (Sclerotium Poriae Cocos)
mix-fried *Gan Cao* (Radix Glycyrrhizae Uralanesis)
Huang Qi (Radix Astragali Membranacei)
Rou Gui (Cortex Cinnamomi Cassiae)
Chen Pi (Pericarpium Citri Reticulatae)
Wu Wei Zi (Fructus Schisandrae Chinensis)
Yuan Zhi (Radix Polygalae Tenuifoliae)
Sheng Jiang (uncooked Rhizoma Zingiberis Officinalis)
Da Zao (Fructus Zizyphi Jujubae)

Formula rationale:

Bai Shao, Chuan Xiong, Dang Gui, and *Shu Di Huang* make up the formula *Si Wu Tang* (Four Materials Decoction) which is the classic formula for nourishing and quickening the blood. *Ren Shen, Bai Zhu, Fu Ling*, and mix-fried *Gan Cao* together create the classic formula *Si Jun Zi Tang* (Four Gentlemen Decoction). This formula is the standard formula for supplementing the qi. These two formulas plus *Huang Qi* and *Rou Gui* make up the formula *Shi Quan Da Bu Tang* (Ten [Ingredients] Completely & Greatly Supplementing Decoction). *Huang Qi* supplements the qi in order to transform the blood. *Rou Gui* warms the channels and promotes menstruation. *Chen Pi* rectifies the qi and transforms dampness, thus benefiting the spleen, the latter heaven root of qi and blood engenderment and transformation. *Wu Wei Zi* nourishes yin, quiets the spirit, and secures the essence. *Yuan Zhi* rectifies the qi and quiets the spirit. *Sheng Jiang* warms and harmonizes the spleen and stomach, while *Da Zao* supplements the qi, nourishes the blood, and quiets the spirit.

D. Qi stagnation

The signs and symptoms of this pattern of delayed menstruation are clots within the menstruate, abdominal distention and pain, and purple-colored blood. In addition, the patient may experience irritability, breast distention and tenderness before the menses, a normal tongue, and a bowstring or choppy pulse. The standard formula for this disorder is *Jia Wei Wu Yao Tang* (Added Flavors Lindera Decoction). This formula courses the liver and resolves depression, quickens the blood and regulates menstruation:

Wu Yao (Radix Linderae Strychnifoliae)
Mu Xiang (Radix Aucklandiae Lappae)
Sha Ren (Fructus Amomi)
Xiang Fu (Rhizoma Cyperi Rotundi)
Bing Lang (Semen Arecae Catechu)
Yan Hu Suo (Rhizoma Corydalis Yanhusuo)
Gan Cao (Radix Glycyrrhizae Uralanesis)

Formula rationale:

Within this formula, *Wu Yao* and *Mu Xiang* move the qi and relieve pain. *Sha Ren* moves the qi, fortifies the spleen, and harmonizes the stomach. *Xiang Fu* courses the liver and rectifies the qi, resolves depression and regulates menstruation. *Bing Lang* rectifies the qi and disperses stagnation. *Yan Hu Suo* moves the qi within the blood and relieves pain. *Gan Cao* harmonizes all the other ingredients in the formula.

Modifications:

Dang Gui (Radix Angelicae Sinensis) and *Chuan Xiong* (Radix Ligustici Wallichii) may be added to the formula to nourish and move the blood.

3. Erratic menstruation

Menstruation that comes with an irregular cycle, sometimes early and sometimes late, is considered "without fixed schedule" or erratic. It is important to note that if the menses come consistently early or consistently late, they fall into the categories of early or delayed menstruation. When the menses are unpredictable in cycle, they are erratic. Such irregularity of the cycle is always related to the liver and kidneys because it is the flow of blood and essence that gives rise to the menstrual periods. Factors such as emotional stress or overwork can lead to binding depression of the liver qi and kidney yin and yang vacuity. Both of these disease mechanisms may lead to obstruction in the vessels or depletion of the blood. Therefore, the two patterns associated with erratic menstruation are binding depression of the liver qi and kidney vacuity.

A. Liver depression qi stagnation

The specific signs and symptoms of liver depression qi stagnation are alternating heavy and light flow of blood with clots in the menstruate, premenstrual breast tenderness, and lower abdominal distention. The patient may also have rib-side pain, headache, a bitter taste in the mouth, reduced appetite, a pale red tongue, and a bowstring, fine pulse. The formula *Xiao Yao San* (Rambling Powder) has the functions of coursing the liver and rectifying the qi, fortifying the spleen and nourishing the blood. Its ingredients consist of:

Chai Hu (Radix Bupleuri)
Dang Gui (Radix Angelicae Sinensis)
Bai Shao (Radix Albus Paeoniae Lactiflorae)
Bai Zhu (Rhizoma Atractylodis Macrocephalae)
Fu Ling (Sclerotium Poriae Cocos)
Gan Cao (Radix Glycyrrhizae Uralanesis)
Sheng Jiang (uncooked Rhizoma Zingiberis Officinalis)
Bo He (Herba Menthae Haplocalycis)

Formula rationale:

Within this formula, *Chai Hu* courses the liver and rectifies the qi. *Dang Gui* nourishes and quickens the blood. *Bai Shao* nourishes the blood, harmonizes the liver, and constrains yin. *Bai Zhu* fortifies the spleen and supplements the qi, while *Fu Ling* fortifies the spleen and quiets the spirit. *Gan Cao* boosts the qi and harmonizes all the other ingredients in the formula. *Sheng Jiang* warms and harmonizes the spleen and stomach. *Bo He* courses the liver and rectifies the qi, resolves depression and clears heat.

B. Kidney vacuity

Patients with kidney vacuity causing erratic menstruation experience a light blood flow that is light in color and accompanied by low back soreness. Other accompanying symptoms may include light-headedness, tinnitus, urinary frequency at night, soft stools, and a fine, forceless pulse. The standard, traditional formula to treat this pattern of this disorder is *Gu Yin Jian Tang* (Secure Yin Decoction), which supplements and enriches the kidneys (both yin and yang aspects) and regulates and rectifies the thoroughfare and controlling vessels. Its ingredients include:

Ren Shen (Radix Panacis Ginseng)
Shu Di Huang (cooked Radix Rehmanniae Glutinosae)
Shan Yao (Radix Dioscoreae Oppositae)
Shan Zhu Yu (Fructus Corni Officinalis)
Tu Si Zi (Semen Cuscutae Chinensis)
Yuan Zhi (Radix Polygalae Tenuifoliae)
Wu Wei Zi (Fructus Schisandrae Chinensis)
mix-fried *Gan Cao* (Radix Glycyrrhizae Uralanesis)

Formula rationale:

Within this formula, *Ren Shen* strongly supplements the qi, quiets the spirit, and engenders fluids. *Shu Di Huang* nourishes the blood and enriches yin, supplements the kidneys and fosters essence. *Shan Yao* supplements both the spleen and kidney's qi while also engendering fluids. *Shan Zhu Yu* nourishes the liver and enriches yin while regulating menstruation. *Tu Si Zi* supplements and enriches, invigorates and fosters kidney yin, yang, and essence. *Yuan Zhi* and *Wu Wei Zi* both quiet the spirit. *Yuan Zhi* also rectifies the qi. Mix-fried *Gan Cao* supplements the qi and harmonizes all the other ingredients in the formula.

Modifications:

It is possible to add more kidney-supplementing, yang-invigorating medicinals if necessary, such as *Ba Ji Tian* (Radix Morindae Officinalis), *Sha Yuan Zi* (Semen Astragali Complanati), and *Rou Cong Rong* (Herba Cistanchis Deserticolae).

5

Chinese Medical Preparation Before *In Vitro* Fertilization: Males

The process of sperm maturation averages 70-90 days. It is, therefore, very beneficial that the male receive acupuncture and Chinese herbal medicine for at least three months prior to starting the IVF procedure. With the help of Chinese medicine, it is possible to improve the quality and quantity of sperm and improve the overall quality of the semen. This, in turn, increases the chances of creating a healthy and viable embryo as well as assists in a more secure implantation.

In Chinese medicine, there are several disease mechanisms that can affect sperm production and quality, such as kidney yang vacuity, kidney yin vacuity, qi stagnation and blood stasis, and damp heat in the lower burner. Standard, traditional Chinese medicinal formulas used to treat male infertility are discussed later in this chapter.

Clinical protocols:

In my clinic, I consistently use several acupuncture points to support men in preparation for IVF:

Qi Hai (CV 6) and *Guan Yuan* (CV 4) help circulate the qi and blood to the testicles. *Bai Hui* (GV 20) stimulates pituitary gland and hormones. If performing acupuncture treatment on the back, *Xin Shu* (Bl 15), *Ge Shu* (Bl 17), *Gan Shu* (Bl 18), *Pi Shu* (Bl 20), *Shen Shu* (Bl 23), and *Da Chang Shu* (Bl 25) can be used. If there is kidney yang vacuity, add *Zhao Hai* (Ki 6) and *Ming Men* (GV 4). If there is kidney yin vacuity, add *Tai Xi* (Ki 3).

In most cases, men with small testicles and low testosterone levels present patterns of kidney yin and/or yang vacuity. They may also present some spleen qi vacuity along with blood vacuity. Other issues helped through supplementing the kidneys may include non-ejaculation, autoimmunity, low sperm count, low quality sperm, and impaired movement or motility.

1. Kidney yang vacuity

Signs and symptoms of kidney yang vacuity in men with fertility issues include tinnitus, dizziness, low back and knee soreness and limpness, cold lower extremities, long, clear urination, nocturia, a pale tongue with thin, white fur, and a deep, slow pulse. In this case, the treatment principles are to supplement the kidneys and warm the essence using *Bu Jing Zhong Zi Fang* (Supplement the Essence & Plant the Seed Formula):

Huang Qi (Radix Astragali Membranacei)
Dang Gui (Radix Angelicae Sinensis)
Tu Si Zi (Semen Cuscutae Chinensis)
Shu Di Huang (cooked Radix Rehmanniae Glutinosae)
Shan Zhu Yu (Fructus Corni Officinalis)
Ba Ji Tian (Radix Morindae Officinalis)
Bai Zhu (Rhizoma Atractylodis Macrocephalae)
Bai Shao (Radix Albus Paeoniae Lactiflorae)

Formula rationale:

This formula supplements the spleen and kidneys as well as the qi, blood, yang, and essence. It mostly improves the quality of the semen and sperm, but there is also some benefit to the quantity of the sperm. *Huang Qi* supplements the qi, while *Dang Gui* nourishes and quickens the blood. *Tu Si Zi* supplements the kidneys, invigorates yang, and boosts the essence. *Shu Di Huang* and *Shan Zhu Yu* supplement the kidneys, nourish yin, and foster the essence. *Ba Ji Tian* likewise supplements the kidneys, invigorates yang, and boosts the essence. *Bai Zhu* fortifies the spleen and boosts the qi. *Bai Shao* nourishes the blood and harmonizes the liver.

Modifications:

For concomitant spleen qi vacuity and weakness, add *Ren Shen* (Radix

Panacis Ginseng) or *Dang Shen* (Radix Codonopsitis Pilosulae). For more marked kidney yang vacuity, add *Yin Yang Huo* (Herba Epimedii), *Bu Gu Zhi* (Fructus Psoraleae Corylifoliae), and *Lu Jiao* (Cornu Cervi) or *Lu Rong* (Cornu Parvum Cervi). For concomitant qi stagnation, add *Zhi Ke* (Fructus Citri Aurantii) and *Yu Jin* (Tuber Curcumae). For blood stasis, add *Dan Shen* (Radix Salviae Miltiorrhizae). For blood vacuity, add *He Shou Wu* (Radix Polygoni Multiflori), *Gou Qi Zi* (Fructus Lycii Chinensis), and *Huang Jing* (Rhizoma Polygonati). For impotence, add *Sha Yuan Zi* (Semen Astragali Complanati) and *Yang Qi Shi* (Actinolitum). For seminal emission, add *Qian Shi* (Semen Euryales Ferocis), *Wu Wei Zi* (Fructus Schisandrae Chinensis), *Sang Piao Xiao* (Ootheca Mantidis), *Yi Zhi Ren* (Fructus Alpiniae Oxyphyllae), *Jin Ying Zi* (Fructus Rosae Laevigatae), and/or *Hai Piao Xiao* (Os Sepiae Seu Sepiellae).

2. Kidney yin vacuity

The signs and symptoms of kidney yin vacuity include low back soreness and limpness, frequent, scanty, yellow urination, nocturia, restlessness, insomnia, impaired memory, malar flushing in the afternoon and early evening, tinnitus, dizziness, a red tongue with scanty fur, and a fine, rapid pulse. The treatment principles for kidney yin vacuity are to supplement the kidneys and enrich yin with *Yang Jing Zhong Zi Fang* (Nourish the Essence & Plant the Seed Formula):

Huang Jing (Rhizoma Polygonati)
Shu Di Huang (cooked Radix Rehmanniae Glutinosae)
Shan Zhu Yu (Fructus Corni Officinalis)
Tu Si Zi (Semen Cuscutae Chinensis)
Gou Qi Zi (Fructus Lycii Chinensis)
Shan Yao (Radix Dioscoreae Oppositae)
Dan Shen (Radix Salviae Miltiorrhizae)
Bai Shao (Radix Albus Paeoniae Lactiflorae)

Formula rationale:

Yang Jing Zhong Zi Fang mostly improves the quantity of the sperm while still improving some of the quality. Within this formula, *Huang Jing* nourishes yin and fosters essence at the same time it fortifies the spleen and supplements the qi. *Shu Di Huang* and *Shan Zhu Yu* supplement the kidneys, nourish yin, and foster essence. *Tu Si Zi* supplements and invigorates kidney yang. *Gou Qi Zi* nourishes liver blood, enriches kidney yin, and fills the essence. *Shan Yao* supplements the spleen and kidneys and engenders fluids. *Dan Shen* quickens the blood and, therefore, improves blood circulation in the testicles to produce well-formed sperm. It also helps quiet the spirit. *Bai Shao* nourishes the blood and harmonizes the liver.

Modifications:

For qi vacuity, add *Dang Shen* (Radix Codonopsitis Pilosulae) and *Huang Qi* (Radix Astragali Membranacei). For spleen vacuity, add *Fu Ling* (Sclerotium Poriae Cocos) and *Bai Zhu* (Rhizoma Atractylodis Macrocephalae). For qi stagnation, add *Chen Pi* (Pericarpium Citri Reticulatae) or *Sha Ren* (Fructus Amomi). For blood vacuity, add *He Shou Wu* (Radix Polygoni Multiflori). For more severe yin vacuity, add *Nu Zhen Zi* (Fructus Ligustri Lucidi) and *Han Lian Cao* (Herba Ecliptae Prostratae).

3. Qi stagnation & blood stasis

If the patient's diagnosis is seminal duct blockage or varicoceles, the treatment is to course the liver and rectify the qi, quicken the blood and dispel stasis with *Huo Jing Zhong Zi Fang* (Quicken the Essence & Plant the Seed Formula):

Chai Hu (Radix Bupleuri)
Dang Gui (Radix Angelicae Sinensis)
Bai Shao (Radix Albus Paeoniae Lactiflorae)
Bai Zhu (Rhizoma Atractylodis Macrocephalae)
Fu Ling (Sclerotium Poriae Cocos)
Gan Cao (Radix Glycyrrhizae Uralanesis)
Zhi Ke (Fructus Citri Aurantii)
Dan Shen (Radix Salviae Miltiorrhizae)

Formula rationale:

Within this formula, *Dang Gui* nourishes and invigorates the blood. *Bai Shao* nourishes the blood and harmonizes the liver. *Chai Hu* courses the liver and rectifies the qi. *Fu Ling* fortifies the spleen and quiets the spirit. *Bai Zhu* fortifies the spleen and supplements the qi. *Dan Shen* quickens the blood, while *Zhi Ke* moves the qi. Thus these two medicinals work together to disperse the blockage of the blood vessels. *Gan Cao* harmonizes all the other ingredients in the formula.

Modifications:

For more qi stagnation, add *Xiang Fu* (Rhizoma Cyperi Rotundi) and *Yu Jin* (Tuber Curcumae). For more blood stasis, add *Mu Dan Pi* (Cortex Radicis Moutan) and *San Qi* (Radix Notoginseng). For depressive heat, add *Zhi Zi* (Fructus Gardeniae Jasminoidis) and *Jin Yin Hua* (Flos Lonicerae Japonicae). For seminal duct blockage, add *Wang Bu Liu Xing* (Semen Vaccariae Segetalis), *Lu Lu Tong* (Fructus Liquidambaris Taiwaniae), and *Chuan Shan Jia* (Squama Manitis Pentadactylis).

Additional points:

Xue Hai (Sp 10) and *Qu Quan* (Liv 8) to quicken the blood

4. Damp heat blocking & obstructing the lower burner

If the Western medical diagnosis is prostatitis, the accompanying signs and symptoms usually include yellow, burning, difficult urination, painful urination, frequent, urgent but inhibited urination, thick, slimy, yellow fur at the base of the tongue, and a bowstring, slippery, possibly rapid pulse. In that case, the treatment principles are to clear heat and eliminate dampness, and the formula to use is *Qing Re Li Yao Fang* (Clearing Heat & Rectifying Medicinal Formula):

Jin Yin Hua (Flos Lonicerae Japonicae)
Huang Bai (Cortex Phellodendri)
Zhi Ke (Fructus Citri Aurantii)
Che Qian Zi (Semen Plantaginis)
Mu Tong (Caulis Akebiae)
Ze Xie (Rhizoma Alismatis Orientalis)
Zhu Ling (Sclerotium Polypori Umbellati)
Sheng Di Huang (uncooked Radix Rehmanniae Glutinosae)

Formula rationale:

Within this formula, *Jin Yin Hua* clears heat and resolves toxins. *Huang Bai* clears heat and dries dampness. *Zhi Ke* moves the qi and clears and disinhibits damp heat. *Che Qian Zi* percolates dampness and supplements the kidneys. *Mu Tong* slightly clears heat and percolates damp through promoting urination. *Ze Xie* clears heat and drains dampness. *Zhu Ling* is very cold and drains dampness through urination. *Sheng Di Huang* nourishes yin and clears heat. It also prevents attacking and draining from damaging righteous yin.

Modifications:

For accompanying qi vacuity, add *Huang Qi* (Radix Astragali Membranacei). For concomitant qi stagnation, add *Zhi Ke* (Fructus Citri Aurantii) or *Chen Pi* (Pericarpium Citri Reticulatae) and possibly *Hou Po* (Cortex Magnoliae Officinalis). For enduring heat damaging the fluids resulting in yin vacuity, add *Mai Men Dong* (Tuber Ophiopogonis Japonici) and *Xuan Shen* (Radix Scrophulariae Ningpoensis). For more marked heat toxins, add *Bai Hua She She Cao* (Herba Hedyotidis Diffusae) and *Zhi Hua Di Ding* (Herba Violae Yedoensitis Cum Radice).

Additional points:

Yin Ling Quan (Sp 9) to drain dampness, *Feng Long* (St 40) to transform phlegm, *Wai Guan* (TB 5) to regulate the water passageways, and *Qu Chi* (LI 11) to clear heat.

Using laboratory reports for medicinal selection

The above Chinese medical pattern discrimination should be used in conjunction with Western medical laboratory results. Semen analysis reports should especially be reviewed. These reports can be used as another way of choosing which group of medicinals to use. For example:

1. Low volume

Low semen volume suggests the need to supplement and enrich kidney yin and foster the essence. In that case, the following medicinals can be used:

Nu Zhen Zi (Fructus Ligustri Lucidi) and *Han Lian Cao* (Herba Ecliptae Prostratae) to supplement and enrich kidney yin

He Shou Wu (Radix Polygoni Multiflori) to nourishe the blood.

Huang Jing (Rhizoma Polygonati) to foster essence.

Zi He Che (Placenta Hominis) to strongly boost the essence and improve the hormone levels.

Additional points:

Tai Xi (Ki 3) is especially good for engendering fluids. Ear: Kidney, Endocrine

2. Low sperm motility

For low sperm motility, one should use medicinals that supplement and invigorate kidney yang as well as supplement the qi (in descending order with the most effective herbs prioritized):

Ba Ji Tian (Radix Morindae Officinalis)
Xian Mao (Rhizoma Cuculiginis Orchioidis)
Tu Si Zi (Semen Cuscutae Chinensis)
Shan Yuan Zi (Semen Astragali Complanati)
Yin Yang Huo (Herba Epimedii)
Rou Cong Rong (Herba Cistanchis Deserticolae)
Lu Rong (Cornu Parvum Cervi)

Additional points:

Zhao Hai (Ki 6) and *Ming Men* (GV 4) are especially good for supplementing the kidneys and invigorating yang. Ear: Kidney, Endocrine

3. Poor liquefaction

For poor liquefaction, use yin-nourishing medicinals such as:

Shu Di Huang (cooked Radix Rehmanniae Glutinosae)
Mai Men Dong (Tuber Ophiopogonis Japonici)
Tian Men Dong (Tuber Asparagi Cochinensis)
Xuan Shen (Radix Scrophulariae Ningpoensis)

Additional points:

Tai Xi (Ki 3) is helpful to nourish yin. Ear: Kidney, Endocrine

4. Abnormal morphology

For abnormal sperm morphology, use blood-quickening medicinals such as:

Dan Shen (Radix Salviae Miltiorrhizae)
Dang Gui (Radix Angelicae Sinensis)

Additional points:

Qu Quan (Liv 8) to quicken the blood. *Xue Hai* (Sp 10) to quicken the blood. If giving acupuncture treatment on the back, use *Ge Shu* (Bl 17) and *Gan Shu* (Bl 18).

Standard Chinese medicinal formulas

The four main disease mechanisms for male infertility are kidney yin vacuity, kidney yang vacuity, qi stagnation and blood stasis, and phlegm dampness.

1. Kidney yang vacuity

For this pattern of male sterility, the formula *Yu Lin Zhu* ([Create a Baby as Perfect as a] Jade Unicorn Pearls) may be used:

Ren Shen (Radix Panacis Ginseng)
Bai Zhu (Rhizoma Atractylodis Macrocephalae)
Fu Ling (Sclerotium Poriae Cocos)
mix-fried *Gan Cao* (Radix Glycyrrhizae Uralanesis)
Bai Shao (Radix Albus Paeoniae Lactiflorae)
Shu Di Huang (cooked Radix Rehmanniae Glutinosae)
Dang Gui (Radix Angelicae Sinensis)
Chuan Xiong (Radix Ligustici Wallichii)
Tu Si Zi (Semen Cuscutae Chinensis)
Lu Jiao (Cornu Cervi)
Du Zhong (Cortex Eucommiae Ulmoidis)
Chuan Jiao (Pericarpium Zanthoxyli Bungeani)

Formula rationale:

Within this formula, *Ren Shen, Bai Zhu, Fu Ling*, and mix-fried *Gan Cao* make up the classic formula *Si Jun Zi Tang* (Four Gentlemen Decoction) which is the standard formula for supplementing the qi. *Bai Shao, Shu Di Huang, Dang Gui*, and *Chuan Xiong* are known together as *Si Wu Tang* (Four Materials Decoction) which nourishes and quickens the blood. *Tu Si Zi* supplements both kidney yin and yang and fosters the essence. *Lu Jiao* supplements and invigorates kidney yang, nourishes the blood and boosts the essence. *Du Zhong* supplements and invigorates kidney yang as well as nourishes liver blood. *Chuan Jiao* warms the spleen and stomach and rectifies the qi.

Modifications:

For severe kidney yang vacuity, add *Yin Yang Huo* (Herba Epimedii), *Ba Ji Tian* (Radix Morindae Officinalis), and *Rou Cong Rong* (Herba Cistanchis Deserticolae).

2. Kidney yin vacuity

If there is kidney yin vacuity pattern male sterility, the formula *Yang Jing Zhong Yu Tang* (Nourish the Essence & Produce [a Baby as Precious as] Jade Decoction) may be used:

Shu Di Huang (cooked Radix Rehmanniae Glutinosae)
Shan Zhu Yu (Fructus Corni Officinalis)
Bai Shao (Radix Albus Paeoniae Lactiflorae)
Dang Gui (Radix Angelicae Sinensis)

Formula rationale:

Within this formula, *Shu Di Huang* supplements and enriches kidney yin and fosters essence. *Shan Zhu Yu* nourishes liver blood, enriches kidney yin, and secures the essence. *Bai Shao* nourishes the blood and constrains yin, while *Dang Gui* nourishes and quickens the blood.

Modifications:

For liver blood vacuity, add *Gou Qi Zi* (Fructus Lycii Chinensis) and *He Shou Wu* (Radix Polygoni Multiflori). For more marked yin vacuity, add *Nu Zhen Zi* (Fructus Ligustri Lucidi), *Han Lian Cao* (Herba Ecliptae Prostratae), and *Mai Men Dong* (Tuber Ophiopogonis Japonici) or *Sha Shen* (Radix Glehniae Littoralis).

3. Qi stagnation & blood stasis

For qi stagnation and blood stasis pattern male sterility, *Kai Yu Zhong Yu Tang* (Open Depression & Produce [a Baby as Precious as] Jade Decoction) can be used:

Dang Gui (Radix Angelicae Sinensis)
Bai Shao (Radix Albus Paeoniae Lactiflorae)
Mu Dan Pi (Cortex Radicis Moutan)
Xiang Fu (Rhizoma Cyperi Rotundi)
Bai Zhu (Rhizoma Atractylodis Macrocephalae)
Tian Hua Fen (Radix Trichosanthis Kirilowii)

Formula rationale:

Within this formula, *Dang Gui* nourishes and quickens the blood. *Bai Shao* nourishes the blood, emolliates the liver, and constrains yin. *Mu Dan Pi* clears heat and cools and quickens the blood. *Xiang Fu* courses the liver, rectifies the qi, and resolves depression. *Bai Zhu* fortifies the spleen and supplements the qi, and *Tian Hua Fen* clears heat and generates fluids, thus helping promote the transformation and enrichment of yin.

Modifications:

For predominant qi stagnation, add *Zhi Ke* (Fructus Citri Aurantii), *Chuan Lian Zi* (Fructus Meliae Toosendan), and *Qing Pi* (Pericarpium Citri Reticulatae Viride). For predominant blood stasis, add *Dan Shen* (Radix Salviae Miltiorrhizae), *Yan Hu Suo* (Rhizoma Corydalis Yanhusuo), *Chi Shao* (Radix Rubus Paeoniae Lactiflorae), and *Yu Jin* (Tuber Curcumae). If there is blockage of the ejaculatory duct, add *Chuan Shan Jia* (Squama Manitis Pentadactylis) and *Wang Bu Liu Xing* (Semen Vaccariae Segetalis).

4. Phlegm dampness

If there is phlegm dampness pattern male sterility, *Qi Gong Wan* (Open the Uterus Pills) can be used:

Ban Xia (Rhizoma Pinelliae Ternatae)
Chen Pi (Pericarpium Citri Reticulatae)
Fu Ling (Sclerotium Poriae Cocos)
Cang Zhu (Rhizoma Atractylodis)
Xiang Fu (Rhizoma Cyperi Rotundi)
Shen Qu (Massa Medica Fermentata)
Chuan Xiong (Radix Ligustici Wallichii)

Formula rationale:

Within this formula, *Ban Xia* dries dampness and transforms phlegm, softens the hard and scatters nodulations. *Chen Pi* rectifies the qi, dries dampness, and transforms phlegm. *Fu Ling* blandly percolates dampness and promotes urination. *Cang Zhu* aromatically dries dampness and fortifies the spleen. *Xiang Fu* courses the liver and rectifies the qi. If the qi moves, fluids move. *Shen Qu* abducts food and disperses stagnation, while *Chuan Xiong* moves the qi and quickens the blood.

Modifications:

For predominant phlegm, add *Zhe Bei Mu* (Bulbus Fritillariae Thunbergii) and *Dan Nan Xing* (bile-processed Rhizoma Arisaematis). For predominant dampness, add *Qu Mai* (Herba Dianthi), *Zhu Ling* (Sclerotium Polypori Umbellati), *Che Qian Zi* (Semen Plantaginis), and/or *Yi Yi Ren* (Semen Coicis Lachryma-jobi).

6

Chinese Medical Treatment Protocols During *In Vitro* Fertilization

This is the most important stage in the *in vitro* fertilization process for both Western and Chinese medicines. When these two systems of medicine are used in conjunction, the results are greatly improved.

1. Start oral contraceptive pills for IVF

This is done one month prior to the IVF procedure to allow the ovaries to rest and to regulate the hormones. This can be thought of as a fallow field that is not cultivated for a season in order for it to be replenished with nutrients.

During this month, the patient should be supported with acupuncture and the formula *Huo Jing Zhong Zi Fang* (Quicken the Essence & Plant the Seed Formula) which courses the liver and rectifies the qi, quickens the blood and fortifies the spleen, and calms the spirit and relaxes the patient:

Dang Gui (Radix Angelicae Sinensis)
Chai Hu (Radix Bupleuri)
Dan Shen (Radix Salviae Miltiorrhizae)
Bai Shao (Radix Albus Paeoniae Lactiflorae)
Fu Ling (Sclerotium Poriae Cocos)
Bai Zhu (Rhizoma Atractylodis Macrocephalae)
Zhi Ke (Fructus Citri Aurantii)
Gan Cao (Radix Glycyrrhizae Uralanesis)

Points: *Zu San Li* (St 36), *San Yin Jiao* (Sp 6), *Tai Chong* (Liv 3), *He Gu* (LI 4), *Yin Tang* (M-HN-3)

Formula Rationale:

Zu San Li is used to fortify the spleen and supplement the qi. *San Yin Jiao* nourishes the blood and is the intersection point of the spleen, liver, and kidney channels. *Tai Chong* used with *He Gu* is known as the Four Bars or Gates. This combination of points strongly courses the liver and rectifies the qi. *Yin Tang* is used to help relax the patient's mind and emotions.

Modifications:

The practitioner may also add *Xue Hai* (Sp 10) to quicken the blood and *Zi Gong Xue* (M-CA-18) to increase circulation to the ovaries.

2. Stimulation of ovaries for IVF

Two to three days after the menstrual cycle begins, the ovaries are stimulated with Follistim, Gonal-F, and Repronex, which function like FSH and LH in order to produce more follicles. At this same time, Chinese medicine should be used to supplement the kidneys and fortify the spleen, nourish the blood and quiet the spirit. This helps to produce more follicles and thicken the lining of the uterus to prepare for the transfer of embryos. It can also reduce the side effects of the drugs. The recommended formula at this time is *Ding Jing Fang* (Stabilize the Menses Formula):

Dang Gui (Radix Angelicae Sinensis)
Shu Di Huang (cooked Radix Rehmanniae Glutinosae)
Shan Yao (Radix Dioscoreae Oppositae)
Fu Ling (Sclerotium Poriae Cocos)
Tu Si Zi (Semen Cuscutae Chinensis)
Chai Hu (Radix Bupleuri)
Bai Shao (Radix Albus Paeoniae Lactiflorae)
Dang Shen (Radix Codonopsitis Pilosulae)
Ba Ji Tian (Radix Morindae Offficinalis)
mix-fried *Gan Cao* (Radix Glycyrrhizae Uralanesis)

Modifications:

For qi vacuity, add *Huang Qi* (Radix Astragali Membranacei). For spleen vacuity, add *Bai Zhu* (Rhizoma Atractylodis Macrocephalae).

For blood vacuity, add *Gou Qi Zi* (Fructus Lycii Chinensis) and *He Shou Wu* (Radix Polygoni Multiflori). For kidney yin vacuity, add *Shan Zhu Yu* (Fructus Corni Officinalis) and *Nu Zhen Zi* (Fructus Ligustri Lucidi). For kidney yang vacuity, add *Rou Cong Rong* (Herba Cistanchis Deserticolae).

Points: *Zu San Li* (St 36), *San Yin Jiao* (Sp 6), *Tai Chong* (Liv 3), *He Gu* (LI 4), *Tai Xi* (Ki 3), *Yin Tang* (M-HN-3), *Bai Hui* (GV 20), and *Zi Gong Xue* (M-CA-18)

Formula Rationale:

Bai Hui stimulates the pituitary gland, thereby increasing FSH levels and stimulating the ovaries. *Zi Gong Xue* also helps to stimulate the ovaries, produce more follicles, improve egg quality, and thicken the lining of the uterus to improve the implantation of the embryo.

3. Before the transfer of embryos for IVF

Chinese medicine is especially helpful in this stage. It can help slightly dilate the cervical opening in order to more easily transfer the embryo into the uterus. It also helps calm the patient, thereby relaxing the uterus. Therefore, when the transfer is being performed, the patient is less likely to experience cramping and uterine contractions, thus helping the embryo implantation.

The formula *Huo Jing Zhong Zi Fang* (Quicken the Essence & Plant the Seed Formula) should be taken just two times: once the night before the transfer of embryos and, secondly, the morning of the transfer. This formula is used to soothe the liver qi and nourish the heart blood in order to quiet the spirit, and to fortify the spleen and supplement the qi in order to hold the embryo in the uterus. *Huo Jing Zhong Zi Fang* consists of:

Dang Gui (Radix Angelicae Sinensis)
Chai Hu (Radix Bupleuri)
Bai Shao (Radix Albus Paeoniae Lactiflori)
Fu Ling (Sclerotium Poriae Cocos)
Bai Zhu (Rhizoma Atractylodis Macrocephalae)
Zhi Ke (Fructus Citri Aurantii)

Dan Shen (Radix Salviae Miltiorrhizae)
Gan Cao (Radix Glycyrrhizae Uralanesis)

Modifications:

For qi vacuity, add *Dang Shen* (Radix Codonopsitis Pilosulae). For anxiety, add *Suan Zao Ren* (Semen Zizyphi Spinosae).

Points: *Zu San Li* (St 36), *San Yin Jiao* (Sp 6), *Tai Chong* (Liv 3), *He Gu* (LI 4), *Tai Xi* (Ki 3), *Yin Tang* (M-HN-3), *Qi Xue* (Ki 13), *Bai Hui* (GV 20), and *Si Shen Cong* (M-HN-1). Include ear points: *Shen Men*, Kidney, Liver, and Spleen.

Qi Xue loosens the cervical opening to make the embryo transfer easier and increases blood flow to the uterus which thickens the uterine lining, helping the implantation of the embryos. *Si Shen Cong* (along with *Bai Hui*) is used to hold the embryo in the uterus and to quiet the spirit. The ear point *Shen Men* also quiets the spirit and relaxes the patient. The Kidney ear point supplements kidney essence and raises the hormone levels. The Liver and Spleen points soothe the qi and nourish the blood.

4. After the transfer of embryos for IVF

After the transfer of embryos, it is important to assist blood circulation in the uterus, maintain implantation of the embryo, and nourish embryo growth. Relaxing the uterus to prevent uterine contractions that could cause bleeding and miscarriage is also important.

Two different formulas are used at this stage depending on whether the patient presents with more kidney yang or kidney yin vacuity.

A. Kidney yang vacuity

An Tai Fang (Safety Fetus Formula) is used to supplement and strengthen kidney yin and yang, fortify the spleen, supplement the qi and blood, and quiet the spirit:

Tu Si Zi (Semen Cuscutae Chinensis)
Xu Duan (Radix Dipsaci Asperi)
Sang Ji Sheng (Ramulus Sangjisheng)

Shan Zhu Yu (Fructus Corni Officinalis)
Dang Shen (Radix Codonopsitis Pilosulae)
Bai Shao (Radix Albus Paeoniae Lactiflorae)
Gou Qi Zi (Fructus Lycii Chinensis)
Bai Zhu (Rhizoma Atractylodis Macrocephalae)
Gan Cao (Radix Glycyrrhizae Uralanesis)

Formula rationale:

Within this formula, *Tu Si Zi* supplements the kidneys and boosts the essence and is good for women with a small uterus. It can also help thicken the lining of the uterus and nourish the embryo. *Xu Duan* supplements and invigorates kidney yang. *Sang Ji Sheng* supplements and nourishes liver blood and kidney yin. *Shan Zhu Yu* enriches liver and kidney yin and secures the essence. *Dang Shen* supplements the qi in order to hold the embryo in the uterus. *Bai Shao* nourishes blood and yin and harmonizes the liver. *Gou Qi Zi* nourishes the blood. *Bai Zhu* fortifies the spleen and supplements the qi. Lastly, *Gan Cao* fortifies the spleen and supplements the qi at the same time as it harmonizes all the other ingredients in the formula.

B. Kidney yin vacuity

If there is predominant kidney yin vacuity, one should use *Yang Tai Fang* (Nourish the Fetus Formula):

Tu Si Zi (Semen Cuscutae Chinensis)
Shu Di Huang (cooked Radix Rehmanniae Glutinosae)
Shan Zhu Yu (Fructus Corni Officinalis)
Shan Yao (Radix Dioscoreae Oppositae)
Bai Shao (Radix Albus Paeoniae Lactiflorae)
Mai Men Dong (Tuber Ophiopogonis Japonici)
Suan Zao Ren (Semen Zizyphi Spinosae)
Gan Cao (Radix Glycyrrhizae Uralanesis)

Formula rationale:

Within this formula, *Tu Si Zi* supplements and boosts kidney essence, while *Shu Di Huang* nourishes and enriches kidney yin and blood. *Shan Zhu Yu* enriches liver and kidney yin and secures the essence. *Shan Yao* supplements the spleen and kidneys as well as engenders fluids. *Bai Shao* nourishes liver yin and harmonizes the liver. *Bai Shao* also strongly relaxes the muscles to prevent the uterus from contracting. *Mai Men Dong* nourishes heart yin and quiets the spirit to also relax the patient. *Suan Zao Ren* nourishes the heart and quiets the spirit, thus relaxing the patient and preventing uterine contractions and miscarriage, and *Gan Cao* fortifies the spleen and supplements the qi at the same time as it harmonizes all the other ingredients in the formula.

Modifications:

For qi vacuity, add *Huang Qi* (Radix Astragali Membranacei). For blood vacuity, add *He Shou Wu* (Radix Polygoni Multiflori) and *Gou Qi Zi* (Fructus Lycii Chinensis). For spleen vacuity, add *Fu Ling* (Sclerotium Poriae Cocos). For a sinking sensation in the lower abdomen, add *Chai Hu* (Radix Bupleuri) and/or *Sheng Ma* (Rhizoma Cimicifugae). For anxiety, add *Long Yan Rou* (Arillus Euphoriae Longanae).

Points: *Zu San Li* (St 36),* *Tai Xi* (Ki 3),* *Yin Tang* (M-HN-3), *Bai Hui* (GV 20). Ear: Kidney, *Shen Men*, and halfway between the Liver & Spleen

Zu San Li and *Tai Xi* should only be used right after the transfer. After a positive hCG or pregnancy test, these points should be omitted because they can be too stimulating.

An Tai Fang or *Yang Tai Fang* can be used to support the patient throughout her pregnancy. Alternatively, a modified version of *Xiao Yao Fang* (Rambling Formula) can be used if the patient suffers from blood stasis and binding depression of the liver qi. This modified version of *Xiao Yao Fang* includes:

Dang Gui (Radix Angelicae Sinensis)
Chai Hu (Radix Bupleuri)
Bai Shao (Radix Albus Paeoniae Lactiflorae)
Bai Zhu (Rhizoma Atractylodis Macrocephalae)
Fu Ling (Sclerotium Poriae Cocos)
Dang Shen (Radix Codonopsitis Pilosulae)

Shu Di Huang (cooked Radix Rehmanniae Glutinosae)
Chen Pi (Pericarpium Citri Reticulatae)
Suan Zao Ren (Semen Zizyphi Spinosae)
Gan Cao (Radix Glycyrrhizae Uralanesis)

Formula rationale:

This formula helps relax the patient and prevents uterine contractions. *Dang Gui* supplements and gently quickens the blood, while *Chai Hu* both courses the liver and upbears the qi. *Bai Shao* nourishes the blood and harmonizes the liver. *Bai Zhu* fortifies the spleen to help engender the blood and hold the embryo. *Fu Ling* fortifies the spleen and quiets the spirit, and *Gan Cao* harmonizes all the other ingredients in the formula. *Dang Shen* is added to supplement qi to help hold the embryo. *Shu Di Huang* nourishes the blood and supplements kidney essence to nourish the embryo. *Chen Pi* rectifies the qi and transforms dampness, thus preventing *Shu Di Huang* from being too slimy and enriching and, therefore, stagnating. *Suan Zao* is used to further quiet the spirit.

7

Prevention of Miscarriage

In Western medicine, there are three stages to a miscarriage or spontaneous abortion: 1) threatened miscarriage, 2) incomplete miscarriage, and 3) complete miscarriage. The patient may experience any or all of these stages. In threatened miscarriage, there is slight bleeding and lower abdominal cramping. However, the cervix is still closed and, therefore, treatment may prevent the further stages of miscarriage from occurring. In this case, a blood test is required to see if there is a positive and high hCG level to indicate a thriving embryo. If a positive and high hCG level is present, there is an approximately 90% success rate of carrying the fetus to full term. However, a positive hCG level that is low may indicate risk of losing the pregnancy.

Unfortunately, if there is heavy bleeding and more painful cramps, an incomplete miscarriage may be experienced. This requires the gynecologist to perform a D & C (dilatation and curettage). In a complete miscarriage, there is gradually less bleeding and cramping and the cervix eventually closes.

IVF & the prevention of miscarriage: clinical experience

Once the embryo has been fertilized and implanted into the uterus, it is extremely important to prevent miscarriage with IVF patients. Female patients around 40 years old experience a miscarriage rate of nearly 50% with IVF alone. However, with the help of Chinese medicine, the rate of miscarriage can significantly be reduced and the pregnancy can be supported to reach full term.

The most important rule to remember in treating threatened miscarriage with Chinese medicine is not to move the qi too forcefully or quicken the blood. Any medicinals or points with these functions will promote the likelihood of miscarriage. The standard, traditional Chinese medicinal formulas for miscarriage are discussed later in this chapter and are useful for reference. Below are the protocols I have personally found useful in dealing with threatened, incomplete, and complete miscarriage.

The following points can be used in cases of threatened miscarriage:

Bai Hui (GV 20) to lift the qi to hold the embryo
Si Shen Cong (M-HN-1) to quiet the spirit and prevent uterine contractions
Yin Tang (M-HN-3) to quiet the spirit
Ear: *Shen Men* to quiet the spirit, Kidney to boost the essence to nourish the embryo, and halfway between the Liver & Spleen to help produce blood to nourish the embryo

Additional points:

For nausea and vomiting: *Shen Que* (CV 8, moxa only), *Zhong Wan* (CV 12), and *Tian Shu* (St 25)
For bleeding: *Bai Hui* (GV 20, moxa only), *Yin Bai* (Sp 1), *Da Dun* (Liv 1), and *Zu San Li* (St 36)
For back pain: (very mild acupuncture only) *Xin Shu* (Bl 15), *Ge Shu* (Bl 17), *Gan Shu* (Bl 18), *Pi Shu* (Bl 20), and/or *Shen Shu* (Bl 23)

In terms of Chinese medicinal support, my clinical practice has focused on supplementing the kidneys in all cases of threatened miscarriage. First, it is essential to identify if the underlying vacuity is more kidney yin or kidney yang. Formulas for each are listed below with modifications to address the other issues affecting each individual patient's case.

1. Kidney yang vacuity

Use *An Tai Fang* (Safety Fetus Formula):

Tu Si Zi (Semen Cuscutae Chinensis)
Xu Duan (Radix Dipsaci Asperi)
Sang Ji Sheng (Ramulus Sangjisheng)
Shan Zhu Yu (Fructus Corni Officinalis)
Bai Shao (Radix Albus Paeoniae Lactiflorae)

Gou Qi Zi (Fructus Lycii Chinensis)
Dang Shen (Radix Codonopsitis Pilosulae)
Bai Zhu (Rhizoma Atractylodis Macrocephalae)
Gan Cao (Radix Glycyrrhizae Uralanesis)

Modifications:

For qi vacuity, add *Huang Qi* (Radix Astragali Membranacei). For spleen vacuity, add *Shan Yao* (Radix Dioscoreae Oppositae) and *Fu Ling* (Sclerotium Poriae Cocos). For kidney yin vacuity, add *Shu Di Huang* (cooked Radix Rehmanniae Glutinosae) and *Han Lian Cao* (Herba Ecliptae Prostratae). For kidney yang vacuity, add *Bu Gu Zhi* (Fructus Psoraleae Corylifoliae) and *Sha Ren* (Fructus Amomi). For vacuity heat, add *Sheng Di Huang* (uncooked Radix Rehmanniae Glutinosae) and *Mai Men Dong* (Tuber Ophiopogonis Japonici). For replete heat, add *Huang Qin* (Radix Scutellariae Baicalensis). For blood vacuity, add *Shu Di Huang* (cooked Radix Rehmanniae Glutinosae), *Huang Jing* (Rhizoma Polygonati), and *He Shou Wu* (Radix Polygoni Multiflori). For nausea and poor appetite, add *Sha Ren* (Fructus Amomi) and *Chen Pi* (Pericarpium Citri Reticulatae). (Do *not* use *Zhi Ke*, Fructus Citri Aurantii, or *Hou Po*, Cortex Magnoliae Officinalis. These medicinals move the qi and the treatment principles forbid this action when preventing a miscarriage.) For vomiting, add *Sheng Jiang* (uncooked Rhizoma Zingiberis Officinalis) and *Ban Xia* (Rhizoma Pinelliae Ternatae). For bleeding due to cold, add *Ai Ye* (Folium Artemisiae Argyii) or carbonized *Jing Jie Sui* (Herba Seu Flos Schizonepetae Tenuifoliae). For bleeding due to heat, add *Han Lian Cao* (Herba Ecliptae Prostratae) and *Ce Bai Ye* (Cacumen Biotae Orientalis). For abdominal pain, add more *Bai Shao* (Radix Albus Paeoniae Lactiflorae) and *Gan Cao* (Radix Glycyrrhizae Uralanesis). For anxiety, add *Suan Zao Ren* (Semen Zizyphi Spinosae), *Long Yan Rou* (Arillus Euphoriae Longanae), and/or *Wu Wei Zi* (Fructus Schisandrae Chinensis). For diarrhea, add *Fu Ling* (Sclerotium Poriae Cocos) and *Mu Xiang* (Radix Aucklandiae Lappae).

2. Kidney yin vacuity

Use *Yang Tai Fang* (Nourish the Fetus Formula):

Tu Si Zi (Semen Cuscutae Chinensis)
Shu Di Huang (cooked Radix Rehmanniae Glutinosae)

Shan Zhu Yu (Fructus Corni Officinalis)
Shan Yao (Radix Dioscoreae Oppositae)
Bai Shao (Radix Albus Paeoniae Lactiflorae)
Mai Men Dong (Tuber Ophiopogonis Japonici)
Suan Zao Ren (Semen Zizyphi Spinosae)
Gan Cao (Radix Glycyrrhizae Uralanesis)

Modifications:

For qi vacuity, add *Huang Qi* (Radix Astragali Membranacei) and *Dang Shen* (Radix Codonopsitis Pilosulae). For blood vacuity, add *He Shou Wu* (Radix Polygoni Multiflori) and *Gou Qi Zi* (Fructus Lycii Chinensis). For spleen vacuity, add *Fu Ling* (Sclerotium Poriae Cocos). For bleeding due to vacuity heat, add *Han Lian Cao* (Herba Ecliptae Prostratae). For bleeding due to replete heat, add *Huang Qin* (Radix Scutellariae Baicalensis). For a sinking sensation in the lower abdomen, add *Huang Qi* (Radix Astragali Membranacei), *Chai Hu* (Radix Bupleuri), and/or *Sheng Ma* (Rhizoma Cimicifugae). For anxiety, add *Long Yan Rou* (Arillus Euphoriae Longanae) and *Wu Wei Zi* (Fructus Schisandrae Chinensis). For low back pain, add *Sang Ji Sheng* (Ramulus Sangjisheng). For insomnia, add *Bai Zhi Ren* (Semen Biotae Orientalis). For nausea, add *Sha Ren* (Fructus Amomi) or *Chen Pi* (Pericarpium Citri Reticulatae). For vomiting, add *Ban Xia* (Rhizoma Pinelliae Ternatae) and/or *Sheng Jiang* (uncooked Rhizoma Zingiberis Officinalis). For abdominal cramps, increase the dosage of *Bai Shao* (Radix Albus Paeoniae Lactiflorae). For headaches, add *Tian Ma* (Rhizoma Gastrodiae Elatae).

Standard formulas:

Traditionally in Chinese medicine, there are four disease mechanisms that may cause miscarriage. They are qi and blood vacuity, kidney qi vacuity, blood heat, and traumatic injury.

1. Qi & blood vacuity

The signs and symptoms are bleeding and a dropping or sinking sensation in the lower abdomen. This may be treated with the classic formula, *Tai Yuan Yin* (Fetal Source Beverage):

Ren Shen (Radix Panacis Ginseng)
Bai Zhu (Rhizoma Atractylodis Macrocephalae)
Dang Gui (Radix Angelicae Sinensis)
Shu Di Huang (cooked Radix Rehmanniae Glutinosae)
Chen Pi (Pericarpium Citri Reticulatae)
Du Zhong (Cortex Eucommiae Ulmoidis)
mix-fried *Gan Cao* (Radix Glycyrrhizae Uralanesis)

Formula rationale:

Within this formula, *Ren Shen* fortifies the spleen, supplements the qi, and quiets the spirit. *Bai Zhu* fortifies the spleen, supplements the qi, and quiets the fetus. *Dang Gui* nourishes the blood. *Shu Di Huang* supplements the liver and kidneys and nourishes yin, blood, and essence. *Chen Pi* rectifies qi and downbears turbidity, thus reflexively promoting upbearing of the clear. It also helps prevent *Shu Di Huang*'s sliminess and enrichment from causing stagnation since it transforms dampness. *Du Zhong* supplements and invigorates kidney yang and quiets the fetus. Mix-fried *Gan Cao* supplements the qi and harmonizes all the other ingredients in the formula.

Modifications:

For severe qi vacuity, add *Huang Qi* (Radix Astragali Membranacei). For spleen vacuity, add *Fu Ling* (Sclerotium Poriae Cocos) and *Shan Yao* (Radix Dioscoreae Oppositae). For blood vacuity, add *Gou Qi Zi* (Fructus Lycii Chinensis) and *He Shou Wu* (Radix Polygoni Multiflori). For kidney yin vacuity, add *Shan Zhu Yu* (Fructus Corni Officinalis) and *Sang Shen Zi* (Fructus Mori Albi). For kidney yang vacuity, add *Xu Duan* (Radix Dipsaci Asperi) and *Bu Gu Zhi* (Fructus Psoraleae Corylifoliae). For kidney yin and yang vacuity, add *Tu Si Zi* (Semen Cuscutae Chinensis) and *Sha Yuan Zi* (Semen Astragali Complanati). For nausea, add *Sha Ren* (Fructus Amomi). For vomiting, add *Ban Xia* (Rhizoma Pinelliae Ternatae) and/or *Sheng Jiang* (uncooked Rhizoma Zingiberis Officinalis). For bleeding, add *Han Lian Cao* (Herba Ecliptae Prostratae) if due to heat or *Ai Ye* (Folium Artemisiae Argyii) if due to cold.

2. Kidney qi vacuity

When kidney qi is unable to hold the fetus, there is low back pain as well as a sinking sensation in the lower abdomen. Other signs and symptoms include vaginal bleeding during pregnancy, dizziness, weak legs, frequent urination, a pale tongue with white fur, and a weak pulse in the cubit position. When the kidneys are insufficient, the thoroughfare and controlling vessels become insecure and malnourished which deprives the fetus of proper nourishment. This leads to restless fetus stirring which, in severe cases, can manifest as vaginal bleeding, a sinking sensation, and sometimes miscarriage. The standard traditional formula given to treat these symptoms is *Shou Tai Wan* (Long Life Fetus Pills). The medicinals in this formula secure the kidneys and quiet the fetus:

Tu Si Zi (Semen Cuscutae Chinensis)
Sang Ji Sheng (Ramulus Sangjisheng)
Xu Duan (Radix Dipsaci Asperi)
E Jiao (Gelatinum Corii Asini)

Formula rationale:

Within this formula, *Tu Si Zi* supplements the kidneys, enriches yin, invigorates yang, and boosts the essence. *Sang Ji Sheng* nourishes liver blood and supplements kidney yin while also specifically strengthening the low back. *Xu Duan* supplements and invigorates kidney yang, strengthens the low back and quiets the fetus. *E Jiao* nourishes the blood, enriches yin, and stops bleeding.

Modifications:

For qi vacuity, add *Dang Shen* (Radix Codonopsitis Pilosulae) and/or *Huang Qi* (Radix Astragali Membranacei). For spleen vacuity, add *Bai Zhu* (Rhizoma Atractylodis Macrocephalae) and *Shan Yao* (Radix Dioscoreae Oppositae). For kidney yin vacuity, add *Shan Zhu Yu* (Fructus Corni Officinalis) and *Shu Di Huang* (cooked Radix Rehmanniae Glutinosae). For kidney yang vacuity, add *Bu Gu Zi* (Fructus Psoraleae Corylifoliae) and *Du Zhong* (Cortex Eucommiae Ulmoidis). For blood vacuity, add *He Shou Wu* (Radix Polygoni Multiflori), *Gou Qi Zi* (Fructus Lycii Chinensis), and *Huang Jing* (Rhizoma Polygonati). For cramps due to uterine contractions, add *Bai Shao* (Radix Albus Paeoneae Lactiflorae) and mix-fried *Gan Cao*

(Radix Glycyrrhizae Uralanesis). For nausea, add *Chen Pi* (Pericarpium Citri Reticulatae) or *Sha Ren* (Fructus Amomi). For vomiting, add *Sheng Jiang* (uncooked Rhizoma Zingiberis Officinalis) and/or *Ban Xia* (Rhizoma Pinelliae Ternatae). For bleeding due to cold, add *Ai Ye* (Folium Artemisiae Argyii) or carbonized *Jing Jie Sui* (Herba Seu Flos Schizonepetae Tenuifoliae). For bleeding due to vacuity heat, add *Han Lian Cao* (Herba Ecliptae Prostratae). For bleeding due to replete heat, add *Huang Qin* (Radix Scutellariae Baicalensis), *Ce Bai Ye* (Cacumen Biotae Orientalis), and *Di Yu* (Radix Sanguisorbae Officinalis).

3. Blood heat

The signs and symptoms of this condition are bright red blood, a red facial complexion, possible low back pain, a red tongue with thick, possibly slimy, yellow fur, and a forceful, rapid pulse. The standard traditional formula for this pattern of threatened miscarriage is *Bao Yin Jian* (Protect Yin Beverage). The medicinals in this formula clear heat, stop bleeding, and nourish the embryo:

Sheng Di Huang (uncooked Radix Rehmanniae Glutinosae)
Huang Qin (Radix Scutellariae Baicalensis)
Huang Bai (Cortex Phellodendri)
Shan Yao (Radix Dioscoreae Oppositae)
Bai Shao (Radix Albus Paeoniae Lactiflorae)
Xu Duan (Radix Dipsaci Asperi)
Gan Cao (Radix Glycyrrhizae Uralanesis)

Formula rationale:

Sheng Di Huang nourishes yin, cools the blood, and stops bleeding. *Huang Qin* clears heat and quiets the fetus. *Huang Bai* also clears heat. *Shan Yao* supplements the spleen and kidneys and engenders fluids. *Bai Shao* nourishes yin, emolliates the liver, and relaxes uterine muscles to prevent uterine contractions and relieve cramps. *Xu Duan* supplements and invigorates kidney yang, strengthens the low back and quiets the fetus. *Gan Cao* harmonizes all the other ingredients in the formula.

Modifications:

For yin vacuity, add *Mai Men Dong* (Tuber Ophiopogonis Japonici). For blood vacuity, add *He Shou Wu* (Radix Polygoni Multiflori) and *Huang Jing* (Rhizoma Polygonati). For low back pain, add *Sang Ji Sheng* (Ramulus Sangjisheng). For bleeding, add *Han Lian Cao* (Herba Ecliptae Prostratae), *Di Yu* (Radix Sanguisorbae Officinalis), and/or *Ce Bai Ye* (Cacumen Biotae Orientalis). For insomnia, add *Suan Zao Ren* (Semen Zizyphi Spinosae) and *Wu Wei Zi* (Fructus Schisandrae Chinensis).

4. Traumatic injury

Any accidents, falls, impacts, or pain-causing conditions may threaten the pregnancy and traditionally are treated with *Sheng Yu Tang* (Sagely Healing Decoction). This famous standard formula supplements the qi, nourishes the blood, and invigorates the kidneys. Even in the case of traumatic injury, it is important not to move the qi too forcefully or quicken the blood during pregnancy so as to prevent miscarriage. *Sheng Yu Tang* secures the fetus, especially if the patient experiences a constant ache in the lower abdomen, has a pale complexion and tongue, is lethargic and withdrawn, and has a fine, weak pulse. It consists of:

Shu Di Huang (cooked Radix Rehmanniae Glutinosae)
Dang Gui (Radix Angelicae Sinensis)
Ren Shen (Radix Panacis Ginseng)
Huang Qi (Radix Astragali Membranacei)
Tu Si Zi (Semen Cuscutae Chinensis)
Sang Ji Sheng (Ramulus Sangjisheng)
Xu Duan (Radix Dipsaci Asperi)

Formula rationale:

Within this formula, *Shu Di Huang* nourishes blood, nourishes and enriches liver and kidney yin, and fosters essence. *Dang Gui* nourishes the blood. *Ren Shen* fortifies the spleen, boosts the qi, and quiets the spirit. *Huang Qi* greatly supplements the qi in order to nourish the blood. *Tu Si Zi* supplements kidney yin, yang, and essence. *Sang Ji Sheng* nourishes and enriches liver blood and kidney yin while also quieting the fetus. *Xu Duan* supplements and invigorates kidney yang, strengthens the low back and quiets the fetus.

Modifications:

For spleen vacuity, add *Bai Zhu* (Rhizoma Atractylodis Macrocephalae) and *Shan Yao* (Radix Dioscoreae Oppositae). For kidney yin vacuity, add *Shan Zhu Yu* (Fructus Corni Officinalis). For kidney yang vacuity, add *Du Zhong* (Cortex Eucommiae Ulmoidis) and *Bu Gu Zhi* (Fructus Psoraleae Corylifoliae). For blood vacuity, add *He Shou Wu* (Radix Polygoni Multiflori) and *Gou Qi Zi* (Fructus Lycii Chinensis). For nausea, add *Chen Pi* (Pericarpium Citri Reticulatae) or *Sha Ren* (Fructus Amomi). For a sinking sensation in the lower abdomen, add *Chai Hu* (Radix Bupleuri) and/or *Sheng Ma* (Rhizoma Cimicifugae). For bleeding due to vacuity heat, add *Han Lian Cao* (Herba Ecliptae Prostratae). For bleeding due to replete heat, add *Ce Bai Ye* (Cacumen Biotae Orientalis) and *Di Yu* (Radix Sanguisorbae Officinalis). For bleeding with cold due to yang vacuity, add *Ai Ye* (Folium Artemisiae Argyii) or carbonized *Jing Jie Sui* (Herba Seu Flos Schizonepetae Tenuifoliae). For abdominal pain, add *Bai Shao* (Radix Albus Paeoniae Lactiflorae) and *Gan Cao* (Radix Glycyrrhizae Uralanesis). For abdominal distention, add *Sha Ren* (Fructus Amomi) or *Chen Pi* (Pericarpium Citri Reticulatae).

8

Case Histories

Case history 1: Irregular menstruation/ premenopause & IVF

Irregular menstruation is one of the symptoms of premenopause. A 48 year-old patient began treatment after receiving a Western medical diagnosis of infertility due to premenopausal syndrome which included irregular menstruation. Her menstrual cycle was 50 days to three months long with heavy bleeding and painful cramping. Therefore, this woman's Chinese medical disease diagnoses were delayed menstruation and painful menstruation and her pattern discrimination was liver blood and kidney vacuity with binding depression of the liver qi. Her signs and symptoms included emotional depression, fatigue, and a pale tongue with white fur. Her pulses were bowstring overall and weak at both cubit positions. Treatment was focused on supplementing the kidneys and boosting the qi, nourishing and quickening liver blood, and coursing the liver and rectifying the qi.

The first step in preparation for IVF was to establish and regulate the patient's menstrual cycle. Before and during her menses, she was given *Xiao Yao Fang* (Rambling Formula), *i.e.*, *Chai Hu* (Radix Bupleuri), *Dang Gui* (Radix Angelicae Sinensis), *Bai Shao* (Radix Albus Paeoniae Lactiflorae), *Bai Zhu* (Rhizoma Atractylodis Macrocephalae), *Fu Ling* (Sclerotium Poriae Cocos), and *Gan Cao* (Radix Glycyrrhizae Uralanesis), to nourish and regulate her cycle. This was modified with *Dan Shen* (Radix Salviae Miltiorrhizae) to quiet the spirit and quicken the blood, *Xiang Fu* (Rhizoma Cyperi Rotundi) to course the liver and rectify the qi, and *Yi Mu Cao* (Herba Leonuri Heterophylli) to quicken the blood, transform stasis, and regulate the menses. *Dang Shen* (Radix Codonopsitis Pilosulae) was added to fortify the spleen and supplement the qi in order to promote both the movement and engenderment of the blood. Acupuncture consisted of the standard prescription of *Zu San Li* (St 36), *San Yin Jiao* (Sp 6), *Tai Xi* (Ki 3), *Tai Chong* (Liv 3), *He Gu* (LI 4), *Yin Tang* (M-HN-3), *Xue Hai* (Sp 10), *Qi Hai* (CV 6), and *Guan Yuan* (CV 4).

Once the patient had completed her next menstrual cycle, she was placed on *Ding Jing Fang* (Stabilize the Menses Formula), *i.e.*, *Dang Gui* (Radix Angelicae Sinensis), *Bai Shao* (Radix Albus Paeoniae Lactiflorae), *Chai Hu* (Radix Bupleuri), *Fu Ling* (Sclerotium Poriae Cocos), *Shan Yao* (Radix Dioscoreae Oppositae), *Dang Shen* (Radix Codonopsitis Pilosulae), *Ba Ji Tian* (Radix Morindae Officinalis), *Tu Si Zi* (Semen Cuscutae), *Shu Di Huang* (cooked Radix Rehmanniae Glutinosae), and mix-fried *Gan Cao* (Radix Glycyrrhizae Uralanesis), to supplement the kidney and spleen qi, nourish the blood, course the liver, and rectify the qi to support ovulation. This prescription was modified with *Gou Qi Zi* (Fructus Lycii Chinensis) to further nourish liver blood and enrich kidney yin. In addition, her acupuncture prescription was altered once her menses were completed by adding *Zi Gong Xue* (M-CA-18) and ear points Kidney and Spleen. *Jian Jing* (GB 21) and *Qu Yuan* (SI 13) were also included for ongoing local neck pain.

After three months of the above treatment, the patient's menstrual cycle was regular with a normal amount of bleeding and only mild cramping. Therefore, during her next attempt at IVF, she was placed on oral contraceptive pills and she began taking *Huo Jing Zhong Zi Fang* (Quicken the Essence & Plant the Seed Formula), *i.e.*, *Dang Gui* (Radix Angelicae Sinensis), *Bai Shao* (Radix Albus Paeoniae Lactiflorae), *Chai Hu* (Radix Bupleuri), *Fu Ling* (Sclerotium Poriae Cocos), *Bai Zhu* (Rhizoma Atractylodis Macrocephalae), *Dan Shen* (Radix Salviae Miltiorrhizae), *Zhi Ke* (Fructus Citri Aurantii), and *Gan Cao* (Radix Glycyrrhizae Uralanesis). This prescription was modified with *Dang Shen* (Radix Codonopsitis Pilosulae) and *Gou Qi Zi* (Fructus Lycii Chinensis) to further supplement qi, blood, and yin. Acupuncture points used at this stage were *Zu San Li* (St 36), *San Yin Jiao* (Sp 6), *Xue Hai* (Sp 10), *Guan Yuan* (CV 4), and *Yin Tang* (M-HN-3).

Once the hormonal stimulation phase began, the patient was placed on

Ding Jing Fang (Stabilize the Menses Formula) once again for its ability to help the body naturally produce more follicles. *Huang Qi* (Radix Astragali Membranacei) was added to supplement qi in order to promote the engenderment and transformation of the blood, while *Shan Zhu Yu* (Fructus Corni Officinalis) was added to supplement and secure the kidney qi. *Gou Qi Zi* (Fructus Lycii Chinensis) was added to nourish the blood and emolliate the liver. Acupuncture treatment consisted of *Zu San Li* (St 36), *San Yin Jiao* (Sp 6), *Tai Chong* (Liv 3), *Tai Xi* (Ki 3), and *He Gu* (LI 4). The Kidney ear point was also included.

Eighteen eggs were produced with the IVF procedure, a very good count considering the patient's age. Unfortunately, during the transfer, the uterine lining was thin at only 0.3cm and the embryos failed to implant. After using acupuncture and Chinese medicinals for another three months, the transfer of her frozen embryos was successful, since the endometrial lining had thickened from 0.3cm to 0.9cm and implantation was able to occur.

Once pregnant, I placed the patient on *An Tai Fang* (Safety Fetus Formula), *i.e.*, *Sang Ji Sheng* (Ramulus Sangjisheng), *Xu Duan* (Radix Dipsaci Asteri), *Tu Si Zi* (Semen Cuscutae Chinensis), *Gou Qi Zi* (Fructus Lycii Chinensis), *Shan Zhu Yu* (Fructus Corni Officinalis), *Dang Shen* (Radix Codonopsitis Pilosulae), *Bai Shao* (Radix Albus Paeoniae Lactiflorae), and *Bai Zhu* (Rhizoma Atractylodis Macrocephalae), for prevention of miscarriage. This formula was modified with the additions of *Huang Qi* (Radix Astragali Membranacei) to encourage holding of the pregnancy by supplementing the qi, and *Shan Yao* (Radix Dioscoreae Oppositae) to supplement both the spleen and kidneys.

The patient now has a healthy six year-old child! Regulating the patient's menstruation and strengthening her ovarian function were key to enabling her to conceive and carry to term.

Case history 2: Decreased ovarian function & IVF

A couple came in for treatment after three failed IVF procedures. The female patient, who was 40 years old, had poor ovarian function and was producing only 1-5 eggs per IVF cycle. Her husband, age 42, had weak sperm. Acupuncture and herbs combined with IVF produced 10 eggs. In their fourth IVF attempt, after treatment with Chinese medicine, the client had produced 10 eggs, became pregnant, and gave birth to a baby girl.

The wife's symptoms included constipation, anxiety, irregular heartbeat, and headaches. Urination was normal. Her pulse was slippery and bowstring, and her tongue was pale with a red tip. Therefore, her Chinese medical pattern discrimination was blood and essence insufficiency with liver-kidney dual vacuity and binding depression of the liver qi. Consequently, my treatment focused on supplementing the kidneys and nourishing the blood, coursing the liver and resolving depression. Vacuity of liver blood and kidney yin is one of the major causes of female infertility in Chinese medicine. The Chinese medical concept of the kidneys correspond directly to the endocrine and reproductive systems. When less blood flows through the reproductive system, less oxygen and nutrients are available to nourish the uterus and ovaries. According to Chinese medical theory, promoting healthy fertility involves improving the circulation of the blood and nutrients to the reproductive system, which is represented primarily by the kidneys.

During administration of birth control pills, the patient was also placed on *Xiao Yao Fang* (Rambling Formula), *i.e.*, *Chai Hu* (Radix Bupleuri), *Dang Gui* (Radix Angelicae Sinensis), *Bai Shao* (Radix Albus Paeoniae Lactiflorae), *Bai Zhu* (Rhizoma Atractylodis Macrocephalae), *Fu Ling* (Sclerotium Poriae Cocos), and *Gan Cao* (Radix Glycyrrhizae Uralanesis) to course the liver and rectify the qi, fortify the spleen and nourish the blood in order to support ovarian function. Her formula was modified with *Dang Shen* (Radix Codonopsitis Pilosulae) to further fortify the spleen and boost the qi, *Tu Si Zi* (Semen Cuscutae Chinensis) and *Ba Ji Tian* (Radix Morindae Officinalis) to supplement the kidneys, invigorate yang, and boost the essence, and *Gou Qi Zi* (Fructus Lycii Chinensis) was added to nourish the blood and emolliate the liver. In addition, the patient was treated with acupuncture points *Zu San Li* (St 36), *San Yin Jiao* (Sp 6), *Tai Xi* (Ki 3), *Tai Chong* (Liv 3), *Zi Gong Xue* (M-CA-18), and *Yin Tang* (M-HN-3). Once this woman stopped taking the oral contraceptive pills, one menstrual cycle passed before the next stage of IVF when acupuncture points *Guan Yuan* (CV 4), *Qi Hai* (CV 6), and *Xue Hai* (Sp 10) were added to her prescription.

The patient began stimulation with Gonal-F at three ampules in the morning and three ampules at night. Then she started Lupron. Once she began hormonal stimulation, all Chinese medicinal prescriptions were stopped at the request of her Western M.D., although acupuncture was continued during her IVF cycle. The patient produced 10 eggs and six embryos for transfer, all of good quality. At this point, acupuncture points *Zu San Li* (St 36), *Tai Xi* (Ki 3), *Tai Chong* (Liv 3), *He Gu* (LI 4), *Zi Gong Xue* (M-CA-18), *Bai Hu* (GV 20), and *Yin Tang* (M-HN-3) as well as ear points Kidney, Spleen, and *Shen Men* were prescribed.

After transfer of the embryos, her acupuncture prescription was changed by removing *Zi Gong Xue* (M-CA-18) so as not to cause additional stimulation to the uterus and adding *Si Shen Cong* (M-HN-1) to quiet the patient's spirit. *Bai Hui* (GV 20) was continued in the prescription in order to upbear the qi and hold the embryos. The procedure was successful, and the patient's daughter is now three years old.

Case history 3: Fallopian tube blockage & IVF

A 42 year-old woman presented with a history of pelvic infections lead-ing to obstruction of her fallopian tubes and infertility. While acupunc-ture and Chinese medicinals alone did not clear this blockage and enable this patient to become pregnant without the use of IVF, the treatments did, however, significantly improve her ovarian function and contributed to the patient's successful IVF procedure. After six months of treatment, the patient produced an unusually large number of follicles with IVF. On average, a woman of her age produces less than 10 follicles in a given IVF cycle. This patient produced 35 folli-cles, 28 eggs, and 21 embryos. These were excellent results. The patient had four transfers before she became pregnant. The first trans-fer of six fresh embryos failed, as well as two consecutive attempts with frozen embryos. Her fourth transfer was successful. In December 2002, she gave birth to healthy twin boys.

This woman's Chinese medical pattern discrimination was liver blood-kidney yin vacuity with qi stagnation and blood stasis. Signs and symp-toms included a pale tongue with teeth-marks on its edges and a red tip, and a bowstring, slippery pulse. She also had painful menstruation and was emotionally irritable. In addition, the woman experienced premenstrual breast distention and pain.

There were two goals of treatment for this patient with acupuncture and Chinese medicinals. First, I addressed the obstruction in her fal-lopian tubes. Second, if she were unable to become pregnant naturally, I prepared her for IVF and pregnancy. In order to improve circulation and remove the obstruction in her fallopian tubes, a modified *Xiao Yao Fang* (Rambling Formula), *i.e.*, *Chai Hu* (Radix Bupleuri), *Dang Gui* (Radix Angelicae Sinensis), *Bai Shao* (Radix Albus Paeoniae Lactiflorae), *Bai Zhu* (Rhizoma Atractylodis Macrocephalae), *Fu Ling* (Sclerotium Poriae Cocos), and *Gan Cao* (Radix Glycyrrhizae Uralanesis), was prescribed. This formula courses the liver, rectifies the qi, and nourishes and quickens the blood. Before her menstruation began, *Suan Zao Ren* (Semen Zizyphi Spinosae), *Gou Qi Zi* (Fructus Lycii Chinensis), *Zhi Ke* (Fructus Citri Aurantii), and *Dan Shen* (Radix Salviae Miltiorrhizae) were added to further course the liver and resolve depression, eliminate vexation and quiet the spirit, quicken the blood and stop pain. Acupuncture points used during the premenstruum were *Zu San Li* (St 36), *San Yin Jiao* (Sp 6), *Xue Hai* (Sp 10), *Tai Xi* (Ki 3), *Tai Chong* (Liv 3), *He Gu* (LI 4), *Guan Yuan* (CV 4), *Qi Hai* (CV 6), and *Zi Gong Xue* (M-CA-18). Ear points Kidney, Spleen, and *Shen Men* were also included. *Xue Hai* (Sp 10) and *Bai Hui* (GV 20) with *Guan Yuan* (CV 4) and *Qi Hai* (CV 6) are a useful combination for increasing hormonal balance as well as for quickening and transforming blood stasis both during and after menstruation.

During her menstrual period itself, the patient was placed on (Menstruation-smoothing Formula), *i.e.*, *Dang Gui* (Radix Angelicae Sinensis), *Bai Shao* (Radix Albus Paeoniae Lactiflorae), *Shu Di Huang* (cooked Radix Rehmanniae Glutinosae), *Chuan Xiong* (Radix Ligustici Wallichii), *Niu Xi* (Radix Achyranthis Bidentae), *Dan Shen* (Radix Salviae Miltiorrhizae), *Xiang Fu* (Rhizoma Cyperi Rotundi), and *Gou Qi Zi* (Fructus Lycii Chinensis), to nourish the blood and emolliate the liver as well as course the liver and rectify the qi. *Lu Lu Tong* (Fructus Liquidambaris Taiwaniae), which moves the qi, and *Wang Bu Liu Xing* (Semen Vaccariae Segetalis), which quickens the blood, were also added. *Rou Gui* (Cortex Cinnamomi Cassiae) was also added to invigorate yang, while *Suan Zao Ren* (Semen Zizyphi Spinosae) was included to quiet the spirit. The same acupuncture points were used as above as well as infrared heat on her abdomen.

Post-menstruation, *Xiao Yao Fang* (Rambling Formula) was modified with *Dang Shen* (Radix Codonopsitis Pilosulae) to supplement the spleen and boost the qi, *Zhi Ke* (Fructus Citri Aurantii) to harmonize the qi, *Shu Di Huang* (cooked Radix Rehmanniae Glutinosae) to supplement the liver and kidneys, nourish the blood and enrich yin, and *Ba Ji Tian* (Radix Morindae Officinalis) to supplement and invigorate kidney yang. After six months of treatment, the patient was still unable to become pregnant with only acupuncture and herbs. Even so, the treatments had been preparing her for IVF.

When she started the IVF program, she took *Huo Jing Zhong Zi Fang* (Quicken the Essence & Plant the Seed Formula), *i.e.*, *Dang Gui* (Radix Angelicae Sinensis), *Bai Shao* (Radix Albus Paeoniae Lactiflorae), *Chai Hu* (Radix Bupleuri), *Fu Ling* (Sclerotium Poriae Cocos), *Bai Zhu* (Rhizoma Atractylodis Macrocephalae), *Dan Shen*

(Radix Salviae Miltiorrhizae), *Zhi Ke* (Fructus Citri Aurantii), and *Gan Cao* (Radix Glycyrrhizae Uralanesis), while she was taking oral contraceptive pills. This formula was modified with *Dang Shen* (Radix Codonopsitis Pilosulae) to supplement the spleen and boost the qi and *Gou Qi Zi* (Fructus Lycii Chinensis) to supplement the liver and nourish the blood. Acupuncture points *Zu San Li* (St 36), *San Yin Jiao* (Sp 6), *Xue Hai* (Sp 10), *Tai Xi* (Ki 3), *Tai Chong* (Liv 3), *He Gu* (LI 4), *Guan Yuan* (CV 4), and *Qi Hai* (CV 6) were needled and infrared heat was used on her abdomen.

Once stimulation began for follicular development, she was placed on *Ding Jing Fang* (Stabilize the Menses Formula), *i.e.*, *Dang Gui* (Radix Angelicae Sinensis), *Bai Shao* (Radix Albus Paeoniae Lactiflorae), *Chai Hu* (Radix Bupleuri), *Fu Ling* (Sclerotium Poriae Cocos), *Shan Yao* (Radix Dioscoreae Oppositae), *Dang Shen* (Radix Codonopsitis Pilosulae), *Ba Ji Tian* (Radix Morindae Officinalis), *Tu Si Zi* (Semen Cuscutae), *Shu Di Huang* (cooked Radix Rehmanniae Glutinosae), and mix-fried *Gan Cao* (Radix Glycyrrhizae Uralanesis), to supplement the kidneys and spleen, course the liver and rectify the qi, nourish the blood and emolliate the liver. Additional modifications were *Chen Pi* (Pericarpium Citri Reticulatae) to aid digestion and *Gou Qi Zi* (Fructus Lycii Chinensis) to nourish the blood. The formula and its modifications helped stimulate and balance the patient's hormonal response to the Western supplements for IVF.

While transferring embryos, the patient was again placed on *Huo Jing Zhong Zi Fang* (Quicken the Essence & Plant the Seed Formula) plus *Dang Shen* (Radix Codonopsitis Pilosulae) and *Suan Zao Ren* (Semen Zizyphi Spinosae) to further boost the qi and quiet her spirit. Her acupuncture prescription remained the same with the addition of *Zi Gong Xue* (M-CA-18) to benefit the uterus, *Bai Hui* (GV 20) to benefit the secretion of pituitary hormones, and ear points Kidney, Spleen, and *Shen Men*.

After transfer of the embryos, *An Tai Fang* (Safety Fetus Formula), *i.e.*, *Sang Ji Sheng* (Ramulus Sangjisheng), *Xu Duan* (Radix Dipsaci Asteri), *Tu Si Zi* (Semen Cuscutae Chinensis), *Gou Qi Zi* (Fructus Lycii Chinensis), *Shan Zhu Yu* (Fructus Corni Officinalis), *Dang Shen* (Radix Codonopsitis Pilosulae), *Bai Shao* (Radix Albus Paeoniae

Lactiflorae), and *Bai Zhu* (Rhizoma Atractylodis Macrocephalae), was prescribed to protect and encourage implantation. It was modified with the addition of *Huang Qi* (Radix Astragali Membranacei) and *Suan Zao Ren* (Semen Zizyphi Spinosae).

Once I knew the patient had conceived, *An Tai Fang* (Safety Fetus Formula) was continued as the base formula for another seven months in order to prevent miscarriage and encourage healthy development of the fetus. Modifications to this formula during this time included the addition of *Huang Qi* (Radix Astragali Membranacei) and *Dang Shen* (Radix Codonopsitis Pilosulae) to fortify the spleen and supplement the qi, *Suan Zao Ren* (Semen Zizyphi Spinosae) to nourish the blood and quiet the spirit, and *Bai Shao* (Radix Albus Paeoniae Lactiflorae) to nourish blood and relax the uterine muscles to prevent uterine contraction. *Mai Men Dong* (Tuber Ophiopogonis Japonici) was also added to enrich yin. The patient's acupuncture prescription was limited to *Bai Hui* (GV 20), *Yin Tang* (M-HN-3), *Si Shen Cong* (M-HN-1), and ear points Kidney, Spleen, and *Shen Men* to avoid overstimulation and prevent miscarriage.

Case history 4: Endometriosis, uterine myomas & no IVF

A 43 year-old patient who had been diagnosed with infertility due to uterine myomas and endometriosis became pregnant without IVF after using only acupuncture and Chinese medicinals. This patient had uterine myomas in the muscular wall of the uterus as well as in the uterine cavity. These myomas were 4 x 5cm in size. An ovarian cyst, 6.5cm in size, had been surgically removed some years prior to treatment with acupuncture and herbs. Signs and symptoms on initial presentation included fatigue, depression, heart palpitations, poor sleep, and occasional loose stools. The woman's urination was normal, but her tongue was pale and dusky with white fur. She suffered from extremely painful cramps during her menstrual cycles and bled profusely. Her pulse was bowstring, slippery, and weak in the cubit positions. Therefore, this woman's Chinese medical diagnosis was painful and excessively profuse menstruation, while her Chinese medical pattern discrimination was binding qi stagnation and blood stasis with liver blood, kidney yin, and spleen qi vacuities.

I decided that we had to treat this woman's uterine myomas and endometriosis first. To accomplish this, I prescribed the basic ingredients of *Xiao Yao Fang* (Rambling Formula), *i.e.*, *Chai Hu* (Radix Bupleuri), *Dang Gui* (Radix Angelicae Sinensis), *Bai Shao* (Radix Albus Paeoniae Lactiflorae), *Bai Zhu* (Rhizoma Atractylodis Macrocephalae), *Fu Ling* (Sclerotium Poriae Cocos), and *Gan Cao* (Radix Glycyrrhizae Uralanesis). I then modified this formula as the case required. For instance, before her menstruation, *Xiao Yao Fang* was replaced with *Dan Shen* (Radix Salviae Miltiorrhizae) to course the liver and rectify the qi, quicken the blood and transform stasis, while *San Leng* (Rhizoma Sparganii Stoloniferi) and *E Zhu* (Rhizoma Curcumae Ezhu) were added to break the blood and disperse accumulation. *Suan Zao Ren* (Semen Zizyphi Spinosae) and *Long Yan Rou* (Arillus Euphriae Longanae) were used interchangeably for quieting her spirit. *Zhi Ke* (Fructus Citri Aurantii) and *Xiao Hui Xiang* (Fructus Foeniculi Vulgaris) were used to regulate and move the qi and quicken the blood to relieve the symptoms of PMS, such as abdominal distention and flatulence. Acupuncture prior to menstruation included *Zu San Li* (St 36), *San Yin Jiao* (Sp 6), *Xue Hai* (Sp 10), *Tai Chong* (Liv 3), *He Gu* (LI 4), and *Zi Gong Xue* (M-CA-18) with infrared heat on her abdomen as her base treatment. Kidney points were omitted, since needling the kidney channel causes hormonal stimulation which would have adversely effected her myomas.

During her menstruation with very heavy bleeding, *Zhi Ben Fang* (Treat the Root Formula), *i.e.*, *San Qi* (Radix Notoginseng), *Yi Mu Cao* (Herba Leonuri Heterophylli), *Xu Duan* (Radix Dipsaci Asteri), *Dang Shen* (Radix Codonopsitis Pilosulae), *Huang Qi* (Radix Astragali Membranacei), *Shan Zhu Yu* (Fructus Corni Officinalis), and *Bai Zhu* (Rhizoma Atractylodis Macrocephalae), was prescribed. *Zhi Ben Fang* supplements the kidneys and spleen in order to contain the blood and secure the essence and so stop excessive bleeding. The kidneys' treasure the essence from which blood is made, and the spleen engenders and transforms the qi and blood and contains the blood within the vessels. This prescription was modified with *Pu Huang* (Pollen Typhae) and *Wu Ling Zhi* (Excrementum Trogopterori Seu Pteromi) to quicken the blood and dispel stasis, stop bleeding and relieve pain. *Pu Huang* and *Wu Ling Zhi* make up an old and popular formula called *Shi Xiao San* (Loose a Smile Powder). It is said that a patient with bad menstrual cramping will suddenly break into a smile of relief when taking *Shi Xiao San*. *Han Lian Cao* (Herba Ecliptae Prostratae) was also added to clear heat and stop bleeding. If the patient's menstruation was only slightly heavy and her cramping was less, *Xiao Yao Fang* (Rambling Formula) was used as the base prescription. This formula was then modified by the addition of *Yi Mu Cao* (Herba Leonrui Heterophylli) to cause her uterus to contract and stop excessive bleeding as well as *San Qi* (Radix Notoginseng), *Pu Huang* (Pollen Typhae), and *Wu Ling Zhi* (Excrementum Trogopterori Seu Pteromi) to quicken the blood, stop bleeding, and relieve pain. During menstruation, the same basic points as during the premenstruum were used with the addition of *Zhong Ji* (CV 3) and *Qi Hai* (CV 6) to reduce cramping. Infrared heat was applied to her abdomen, while moxibustion was used on *Bai Hui* (GV 20), *Da Dun* (Liv 1), *Yin Bai* (Sp 1), and *Zu San Li* (St 36) to promote containment of the blood and to stop bleeding. After menstruation, the woman was treated with the same base prescription plus *Qu Quan* (Liv 8) to both nourish the liver as well as move stagnation. *Zi Gong Xue* (M-CA-18) was also added to increase circulation in the uterus and treat the myomas. Ear points Kidney, Spleen, and *Shen Men* were added as well as *Bai Hui* (GV 20) to encourage pregnancy. Infrared heat was also used. After just a little over six months of Chinese medical treatment, this woman's menstrual bleeding was normal in amount and the severe cramping had been alleviated.

When Western medical examination showed that this woman's uterine myomas were under control, treatment refocused on preparing the patient for pregnancy. *Xiao Yao Fang* (Rambling Powder) was again used as the base formula with modifications to encourage conception. The patient quickly became pregnant. However, years of heavy bleeding had caused the patient to have a blood vacuity. Therefore, supplementing medicinals were added to *Xiao Yao Fang*, such as *Shu Di Huang* (cooked Radix Rehmanniae Glutinosae) and *Gou Qi Zi* (Fructus Lycii Chinensis) to supplement liver blood and enrich kidney yin and *Dang Shen* (Radix Codonopsitis Pilosulae) to supplement the spleen and boost the qi so as to promote the spleen's functions of containing the blood within the vessels and increasing engenderment of new blood. *Dan Shen* (Radix Salviae Miltiorrhizae) and *Zhi Ke* (Fructus Citri Aurantii) were added to quicken the blood and move the qi respectively. *Nu Zhen Zi* was added to supplement the kidneys and nourish yin. *San Leng* (Rhizoma Sparganii Stoloniferi), *E Zhu* (Rhizoma Curcumae Ezhu), and *Tao Ren* (Semen Pruni Persciae) were added to quicken the blood and transform stasis to continue addressing the stagnation due to the myomas.

Unfortunately, because uterine myomas are estrogen sensitive, the hormone stimulation of pregnancy caused her myomas to begin growing again. She had a brief period of spotting in the first six weeks of pregnancy which I addressed with acupuncture and herbs. Then, in the fifth month of pregnancy, when the myomas had increased to 6 x 4cm in size, the additional stress in her uterus caused uterine contractions which threatened the pregnancy. The patient's uterus was contracting painfully at least 10 times per day. Her cervix opened an inch in diameter, and she began spotting and passing clots. After Western medical evaluation, the patient was informed she must prepare for imminent delivery and possible loss of the fetus. Instead, the patient turned to Chinese medicine for an alternative to delivery of such an early pregnancy.

During the first six weeks of her pregnancy, when the patient had light spotting, she was placed on *An Tai Fang* (Safety Fetus Formula), *i.e.,* *Sang Ji Sheng* (Ramulus Sangjisheng), *Xu Duan* (Radix Dipsaci Asteri), *Tu Si Zi* (Semen Cuscutae Chinensis), *Gou Qi Zi* (Fructus Lycii Chinensis), *Shan Zhu Yu* (Fructus Corni Officinalis), *Dang Shen* (Radix Codonopsitis Pilosulae), *Bai Shao* (Radix Albus Paeoniae Lactiflorae), and *Bai Zhu* (Rhizoma Atractylodis Macrocephalae). This formula was modified with *Sha Yuan Zi* (Semen Astragali Complanati) to supplement the kidneys and secure the essence and *Huang Qi* (Radix Astragali Membranacei) to fortify the spleen and boost the qi, thus helping to prevent miscarriage. *Fu Ling* (Sclerotiun Poria Cocos) was combined with *Shan Yao* (Radix Dioscoreae Oppositae) to also supplement the kidneys and spleen and thus strengthen both the former and latter heaven roots of the patient. *Shu Di Huang* (cooked Radix Rehmanniae Glutinosae) was added to nourish liver blood and foster kidney essence, while *Han Lian Cao* (Herba Ecliptae Prostratae) was added to enrich yin, clear heat, and stop bleeding. For nausea and loose stools in early pregnancy, *Chen Pi* (Pericarpium Citri Reticulatae), *Mai Ya* (Fructus Germinatus Hordei Vulgaris), and *Wu Wei Zi* (Fructus Schisandrae Chinensis) were included along with *Sha Ren* (Fructus Amomi) to specifically harmonize the stomach, downbear counterflow, and quiet the fetus.

In the fifth month, when the patient began contractions due to the increase in size of the myomas described above, *An Tai Fang* (Safety Fetus Formula) was modified with a large dosage of *Bai Shao* (Radix Albus Paeoniae Lactiflorae) and *Gan Cao* (Radix Glycyrrhizae Uralanesis). *Bai Shao* and *Gan Cao* make up a famous prescription *Shao Yao Gan Cao Tang* (Peony & Licorice Decoction) first mentioned in the classic text, the *Shang Han Lun (The Treatise on Damage [Due to] Cold)*, for stopping spasms and alleviating pain. Here, this pair were used to alleviate uterine contractions. *Sha Ren* (Fructus Amomi) was added to rectify the qi. *Sha Ren* has a special function of moving and rectifying the qi while not injuring the fetus. Most qi-moving medicinals are used with great care during pregnancy, but *Sha Ren* is a safe choice. *Suan Zao Ren* (Semen Zizyphi Spinosae) and *Mai Men Dong* (Tuber Ophiopogonis Japonici) were added to reduce anxiety and help the patient rest at night as well as enrich yin. Once pregnant, only *Bai Hui* (GV 20) and *Yin Tang* (M-HN-3) were needled along with ear points Kidney, Spleen, and *Shen Men* to prevent miscarriage. (Please note that although kidney channel points are not used when myomas are present, the use of the Kidney ear point was used because the need to prevent miscarriage was more important at this stage.) Infrared heat was also used on the patient's feet, to gently stimulate *Da Dun* (Liv 1) and *Yin Bai* (Sp 1) to prevent bleeding and miscarriage.

Acupuncture and Chinese medicinals enabled the patient to maintain her pregnancy, carry to full term, and give birth to a healthy baby boy.

Case history 5: Infertility, male & female, and treatment after IVF

A 37 year-old woman came in for treatment with the Western medical diagnosis of infertility. She and her husband had been trying to conceive for four years prior to coming to my clinic. She had two failed IVF attempts and three failed intrauterine inseminations (IUIs) before treatment with acupuncture and Chinese medicinals. In her previous IVF cycles, only 2-7 follicles were produced. This demonstrated poor ovarian function. Her husband's sperm was reported to be of poor quality, with a motility of 14% (normal is >50%) and a total count of 0.6 m/ml (normal is >25 m/ml). Therefore, I treated both the husband and the wife with acupuncture and herbs.

The third IVF, which took place two months into receiving acupuncture and herbs in my clinic, also produced only three follicles. Because of this, the third attempt at IVF was abandoned. Instead, the patient used IUI. While she did not become pregnant in the procedure, the patient did conceive one month later on a natural cycle without the use of IVF or IUI. The hormones used in IVF linger for over a month and continue to influence a woman's ovarian function. I would encourage women to keep this in mind and to not give up after the disappointment of a failed IVF. This case was an example of how important it is to continue trying to get pregnant in the months after an IVF cycle.

Treatment was focused on the patient's Chinese medical pattern discrimination of kidney vacuity with qi stagnation and blood stasis. This woman's presenting signs and symptoms were fatigue, tinnitus, poor sleep, vaginal dryness, and low sex drive for several years. She was emotionally depressed. She also experienced discomfort in her lower abdomen and very bad cramps at the beginning of her menstrual cycle. Her tongue was slightly dusky with white fur and a red tip, while her pulse was weak in both cubit positions and slippery overall.

In preparation for IVF, the patient was placed on *Xiao Yao Fang* (Rambling Formula), *i.e.*, *Chai Hu* (Radix Bupleuri), *Dang Gui* (Radix Angelicae Sinensis), *Bai Shao* (Radix Albus Paeoniae Lactiflorae), *Bai Zhu* (Rhizoma Atractylodis Macrocephalae), *Fu Ling* (Sclerotium Poriae Cocos), and *Gan Cao* (Radix Glycyrrhizae Uralanesis), before and during her menstruation to course the liver and rectify the qi as well as nourish the blood. This was modified with *Dang Shen* (Radix Codonopsitis Pilosulae) to fortify the spleen and supplement the qi and *Zhi Ke* (Fructus Citri Aurantii) to further regulate and rectify the qi. After her menstruation, she was placed on *Ding Jing Fang* (Stabilize the Menses Formula), *i.e.*, *Dang Gui* (Radix Angelicae Sinensis), *Bai Shao* (Radix Albus Paeoniae Lactiflorae), *Chai Hu* (Radix Bupleuri), *Fu Ling* (Sclerotium Poriae Cocos), *Shan Yao* (Radix Dioscoreae Oppositae), *Dang Shen* (Radix Codonopsitis Pilosulae), *Ba Ji Tian* (Radix Morindae Officinalis), and mix-fried *Gan Cao* (Radix Glycyrrhizae Uralanesis), to supplement the qi and nourish the blood. *Tu Si Zi* (Semen Cuscutae Chinensis) was removed from the base formula and *Sha Yuan Zi* (Semen Astragali Complanati) was added instead to supplement the kidneys and both nourish yin and invigorate yang. *Suan Zao Ren* (Semen Zizyphi Spinosae) was added to nourish the blood and quiet her spirit. *Long Yan Rou* (Arillis Euphoriae Longanae) was chosen as a modification to fortify the spleen and boost the qi, supplement the heart and nourish the blood. *Chen Pi* (Pericarpium Citri Reticulatae) was added to aid digestion. At ovulation, to warm and invigorate yang, even more *Ba Ji Tian* (Radix Morindae Officinalis) and *Zhi Ke* (Fructus Citri Aurantii) were added to relax the cervix, thereby facilitating the sperm's entrance into the uterus. Acupuncture before and during her menses consisted of *Zu San Li* (St 36), *San Yin Jiao* (Sp 6), *Tai Xi* (Ki 3), *Tai Chong* (Liv 3), *He Gu* (LI 4), *Bai Hui* (GV 20), and *Yin Tang* (M-HN-3). *Xue Hai* (SP 10), *Zhong Ji* (CV 3), *Qi Hai* (CV 6) and ear points Kidney, Spleen, and *Shen Men* were also used. Infrared heat was used on her lower abdomen in all treatments. After menstruation, *Xue Hai*, *Zhong Ji*, and *Qi Hai* were removed from the above prescription, and *Zi Gong Xue* (M-CA-18) was added. Heat was again applied with the infrared lamp.

After two months of treatment, the patient's menstruation was less painful with fewer cramps and less clotting. Emotionally, she felt happier and her energy was very much improved. The husband's semen also improved over the course of his treatment. His pulses were small and weak bilaterally in the cubit positions. His tongue was pale with white fur. I categorized his pattern as liver blood and kidney vacuity with some liver depression qi stagnation. Therefore, his herbal prescription was a modified *Xiao Yao Fang* (Rambling Formula).

Modifications included added *Zhi Ke* (Fructus Citri Aurantii) and *Dan Shen* (Radix Salviae Miltiorrhizae) to regulate and rectify the qi and blood, *Dang Shen* (Radix Codonopsitis Pilosulae) to fortify the spleen, supplement the qi, and generate fluids, and *Suan Zao Ren* (Semen Zizyphi Spinosae) to nourish the liver and quiet the spirit. The patient was also treated with acupuncture points *Zu San Li* (St 36), *Tai Chong* (Liv 3), *San Yin Jiao* (Sp 6), *He Gu* (LI 4), *Qi Hai* (CV 6), and *Yin Tang* (M-HN-3) along with infrared heat treatments on his lower abdomen.

While the third IVF attempt was not successful, once the patient's natural cycle returned the following month, she did conceive and carried the baby full term. Once pregnant, her treatment focused on maintaining a healthy pregnancy. Therefore, she was placed on *An Tai Fang* (Safety Fetus Formula), *i.e.*, *Sang Ji Sheng* (Ramulus Sangjisheng), *Xu Duan* (Radix Dipsaci Asteri), *Tu Si Zi* (Semen Cuscutae Chinensis), *Gou Qi Zi* (Fructus Lycii Chinensis), *Shan Zhu Yu* (Fructus Corni Officinalis), *Dang Shen* (Radix Codonopsitis Pilosulae), *Bai Shao* (Radix Albus Paeoniae Lactiflorae), and *Bai Zhu* (Rhizoma Atractylodis Macrocephalae). This was modified with *E Jiao* (Gelatinum Corii Asini) to nourish the blood and prevent bleeding. *Shan Yao* (Radix Dioscoreae Opppositae) was also added to supplement the spleen and kidney qi and yin, and *Gan Cao* (Radix Glycyrrhizae Uralanesis) was added to harmonize all the other medicinals in the prescription. No acupuncture was used once this patient became pregnant, although moxibustion was applied to *Bai Hui* (GV 20) and *Zu San Li* (St 36) as a preventative against miscarriage. The patient now has a healthy three year-old daughter!

Case history 6: Thin endometrial lining & IVF

A 45 year-old woman came to the clinic for infertility. She had a 17 year-old son from a previous marriage and was attempting another pregnancy in her second marriage. Three years previously, she had undergone IVF but had miscarried. Because her husband's semen analysis showed poor semen quality, I also treated the patient's spouse.

The woman's medical history showed light menstrual periods and a thin endometrial lining (4-5mm). Since the miscarriage, she had chronic pelvic infections with lower abdominal pain. The patient experienced low back pain on the right side, headaches, fatigue, loose stools, and emotional lability. Her tongue was pale with white fur and cracks on its surface. Her pulse was slippery and weak in the cubit positions. Based on these signs and symptoms, I categorized the patient's Chinese medical pattern as kidney and blood vacuity with qi stagnation and blood stasis. For six months, the patient prepared for IVF and received different formulas according to her menstrual cycle. Treatment principles were to supplement the kidneys and nourish the blood, course the liver and rectify the qi, quicken the blood and transform stasis.

Accordingly, before menstruation, she took *Xiao Yao Fang* (Rambling Formula), *i.e.*, *Chai Hu* (Radix Bupleuri), *Dang Gui* (Radix Angelicae Sinensis), *Bai Shao* (Radix Albus Paeoniae Lactiflorae), *Bai Zhu* (Rhizoma Atractylodis Macrocephalae), *Fu Ling* (Sclerotium Poriae Cocos), and *Gan Cao* (Radix Glycyrrhizae Uralanesis), which was modified by the addition of *Zhi Ke* (Fructus Citri Aurantii) and *Dan Shen* (Radix Salviae Miltiorrhizae) to rectify and move the qi and blood, and *Shu Di Huang* (cooked Radix Rehmanniae Glutinosae) and *Suan Zao Ren* (Semen Zizyphi Spinosae) to nourish the blood and quiet the spirit. Acupuncture points needled consisted of *Zu San Li* (St 36), *San Yin Jiao* (Sp 6), *Tai Xi* (Ki 3), *Tai Chong* (Liv 3), *He Gu* (LI 4), and *Yin Tang* (M-HN-3). Ear points included Kidney, Spleen, *Shen Men*, and Uterus.

During menstruation, the patient was taken off *Xiao Yao Fang* (Rambling Formula) and was given the following Chinese medicinals: *Shu Di Huang* (cooked Radix Rehmanniae Glutinosae) and *Dang Gui* (Radix Angelicae Sinensis) to nourish the blood, *Chuan Xiong* (Radix

Ligustici Wallichii) to move the qi and quicken the blood, and *Chi Shao* (Radix Rubrus Paeoniae Lactiflorae) to also quicken the blood and dispel stasis. *Gan Jiang* (dry Rhizoma Zingiberis Officinalis) was used to warm and invigorate yang, warm the channels and stop bleeding. *Rou Gui* (Cortex Cinnamomi Cassiae) was used to warm spleen and kidney yang. *Niu Xi* (Radix Achyranthis Bidentatae) and *Dan Shen* (Radix Salviae Miltiorrhizae) were added to further move the qi and quicken the blood, while *Xiao Hui Xiang* (Fructus Foeniculi Vulgaris) was used to rectify the qi and warm the liver channel so as to disperse stagnation and relieve pain. *San Qi* (Radix Notoginseng) was also included to quicken the blood and transform stasis, stop bleeding and relieve pain. Acupuncture body and ear points were the same as before menstruation with the addition of supplementation at the points *Guan Yuan* (CV 4) and *Qi Hai* (CV 6) accompanied by infrared heat.

After menstruation, the patient's medicinals were changed again. At this stage in the cycle, they included: *Huang Qi* (Radix Astragali Membranacei), *Dang Gui* (Radix Angelicae Sinensis), *Tu Si Zi* (Semen Cuscutae Chinensis), *Du Zhong* (Cortex Eucommiae Ulmoidis), *Rou Cong Rong* (Herba Cistanchis Deserticolae), *Suo Yang* (Herba Cynomorii Songarici), *Shu Di Huang* (cooked Radix Rehmanniae Glutinosae), *Bai Shao* (Radix Albus Paeoniae Lactiflorae), *Ba Ji Tian* (Radix Morindae Officinalis), and *Gou Qi Zi* (Fructus Lycii Chinensis). Depending on the patient's symptoms, the following medicinals were added as modifiers: *Sha Yuan Zi* (Semen Astragali Complanati) to supplement the kidneys and thicken the uterine lining, *Zhi Ke* (Fructus Citri Aurantii) to rectify the qi in case of depression, and *Dan Shen* (Radix Salviae Miltiorrhizae) for heart palpitations. *Sang Ji Shen* (Ramulus Sangjisheng) and *Xu Duan* (Radix Dipsaci Asteri) were added to supplement the kidneys and treat low back pain. *Yin Yang Huo* (Herba Epimedii) was included to stimulate the follicles during ovulation. *Fu Ling* (Sclerotium Poriae Cocos) and *Bai Zhu* (Rhizoma Atractylodis Macrocephalae) were used to fortify the spleen and boost the qi in order to reduce loose stools and relieve digestive problems, while *Shan Zhu Yu* (Fructus Corni Officinalis) was included to supplement the kidneys, enrich yin, and thicken the uterine lining. *Chen Pi* (Pericarpium Citri Reticulatae) was added to relieve abdominal distention and flatulence. Modifying herbs were chosen for their specific properties and their applicability to the patient's needs at time of treatment. Acupuncture points at this stage included *Di Ji* (Sp 8), *Tai Xi* (Ki 3), *Zhao Hai* (Ki 6), *Fu Liu* (Ki 7), *Bai Hui* (GV 20), *Zu San Li* (St 36), and *Si Shen Cong* (M-HN-1). Ear points were Kidney, Spleen, and *Shen Men*.

During this time her husband also received treatments to improve the quality of his sperm. By increasing sperm quality and thickening the uterine lining, the chances of a successful implantation were greatly improved. While preparing for IVF, the couple continued to attempt at conceiving naturally, but this was not successful.

IVF treatment involved a donor egg and the husband's sperm. In order to harvest the eggs and transfer the fertilized embryos, oral contraceptive pills were used to synchronize the patient's and the donor's menstrual cycles. The following herbs were given prior to embryo transfer: *Dang Shen* (Radix Codonopsitis Pilosulae) to supplement the qi, *Fu Ling* (Sclerotium Poriae Cocos) and *Bai Zhu* (Rhizoma Atractylodis Macrocephalae) to fortify the spleen, *Chen Pi* (Pericarpium Citri Reticulatae) to rectify the qi and aid digestion, and *Bai Shao* (Radix Albus Paeoniae Lactiflorae) to course the liver, rectify the qi, and relax uterine muscles. *Gou Qi Zi* (Fructus Lycii Chinensis) and *Shu Di Huang* (cooked Radix Rehmanniae Glutinosae) were added to nourish the blood and yin, while *Ba Ji Tian* (Radix Morindae Officinalis) and *Rou Gui* (Cortex Cinnamomi Cassiae) were included to invigorate and warm yang. Lastly, *Gan Cao* (Radix Glycyrrhizae Uralanesis) was included to harmonize all the other medicinals in the prescription and further supplement the qi. Acupuncture points consisted of *Zu San Li* (St 36), *San Yin Jiao* (Sp 6), *Tai Xi* (Ki 3), *Tai Chong* (Liv 3), *He Gu* (LI 4), *Yin Tang* (M-HN-3), *Xue Hai* (Sp 10), and *Zi Gong Xue* (M-CA-18).

When bleeding during menstruation, the patient took *Xiao Yao Fang* (Rambling Powder), *i.e.*, *Chai Hu* (Radix Bupleuri), *Dang Gui* (Radix Angelicae Sinensis), *Bai Shao* (Radix Albus Paeoniae Lactiflorae), *Bai Zhu* (Rhizoma Atractylodis Macrocephalae), *Fu Ling* (Sclerotium Poriae Cocos), and *Gan Cao* (Radix Glycyrrhizae Uralanesis), plus *Dan Shen* (Radix Salviae Miltiorrhizae) and *Xiang Fu* (Rhizoma Cyperi Rotundi) to regulate menstruation, *Gou Qi Zi* (Fructus Lycii Chinensis) to nourish the blood, and *Rou Gui* (Cortex Cinnamomi Cassiae) to warm yang, promote menstruation, and relieve pain.

Acupuncture points needled during menstruation included *Zu San Li* (St 36), *San Yin Jiao* (Sp 6), *Tai Xi* (Ki 3), *Tai Chong* (Liv 3), *He Gu* (LI 4), *Yin Tang* (M-HN-3), *Xue Hai* (Sp 10), *Guan Yuan* (CV 4), and *Qi Hai* (CV 6). The patient's bleeding was normal in quantity and quality, whereas previously it was too light in flow. An ultrasound also showed that the uterine lining was greatly improved, thickening to 10mm, whereas previously it was only 4-5mm. Without an adequate uterine lining, implantation is not likely, and the risk of miscarriage is very high. The increase in the patient's uterine lining was very encouraging and led to a successful pregnancy for this patient.

During the two week period between the end of menstruation and ovulation, the patient continued on *Xiao Yao Fang* (Rambling Formula) but modified with *Suan Zao Ren* (Semen Zizyphi Spinosae), *Dang Shen* (Radix Codonopsitis Pilosulae), *Tu Si Zi* (Semen Cuscutae Chinensis), and *Shan Zhu Yu* (Fructus Corni Officinalis). Acupuncture points needled during this same period were *Zu San Li* (St 36), *San Yin Jiao* (Sp 6), *Tai Xi* (Ki 3), *Tai Chong* (Liv 3), *He Gu* (LI 4), *Yin Tang* (M-HN-3), and *Zi Gong Xue* (M-CA-18). The doner provided four eggs, all of which developed into viable embryos which were available for transfer.

After transfer of the four embryos, the patient experienced nausea, chills, nasal congestion, fatigue, lower abdominal tenderness and aching, and low back soreness. She was also emotionally sensitive and depressed. Therefore, I administered *Liu Jun Zi Fang* (Six Gentlemen Formula), *i.e.*, *Dang Shen* (Radix Codonopsitis Pilosulae), *Fu Ling* (Sclerotium Poriae Cocos), *Bai Zhu* (Rhizoma Atractylodis Macrocephalae), *Ban Xia* (Rhizoma Pinelliae Ternatae), *Chen Pi* (Pericarpium Citri Reticulatae), and *Gan Cao* (Radix Glycyrrhizae Uralanesis), for eliminating nausea. This formula was further modified to improve the success of embryo implantation. Added medicinals included *Huang Qi* (Radix Astragali Membranacei) to supplement the qi and hold the embryo, *Bai Shao* (Radix Albus Paeoniae Lactiflorae) to relax the uterus, *Du Zhong* (Cortex Eucommiae Ulmoidis) to nourish liver blood and quiet the fetus (should implantation occur), and *Gou Qi Zi* (Fructus Lycii Chinensis) to nourish the blood and, therefore, the embryo. Acupuncture points consisted of *Zu San Li* (St 36), *Tai Xi* (Ki 3), *Bai Hui* (GV 20), *Si Shen Cong* (M-HN-1), and *Yin Tang* (M-HN-3). Ear points consisted of Kidney, Spleen, and *Shen Men*.

Implantation and pregnancy proved to be successful. The patient was given 2mg of estradiol and 50mg of progesterone daily to help prevent miscarriage. To complement this, *An Tai Fang* (Safety Fetus Formula), *i.e.*, *Sang Ji Sheng* (Ramulus Sangjisheng), *Xu Duan* (Radix Dipsaci Asteri), *Tu Si Zi* (Semen Cuscutae Chinensis), *Gou Qi Zi* (Fructus Lycii Chinensis), *Shan Zhu Yu* (Fructus Corni Officinalis), *Dang Shen* (Radix Codonopsitis Pilosulae), *Bai Shao* (Radix Albus Paeoniae Lactiflorae), and *Bai Zhu* (Rhizoma Atractylodis Macrocephalae), was prescribed. Modifications included the addition of *Chen Pi* (Pericarpium Citri Reticulatae) for abdominal distention and flatulence and *Gou Qi Zi* (Fructus Lycii Chinensis) to nourish the blood in order to stop heart palpitations. *Ban Xia* (Rhizoma Pinelliae Ternatae) was added for nausea, and *Fu Ling* (Sclerotium Poriae Cocos) was added to quiet the spirit and fortify the spleen. *Huang Qi* (Radix Astragali Membranacei) was included to supplement qi in order to hold the embryo. Acupuncture points treated at this time included *Tai Xi* (Ki 3), *Zu San Li* (St 36), *Bai Hui* (GV 20), *Yin Tang* (M-HN-3), and *Si Shen Cong* (M-HN-1). Ear points Kidney, Spleen, and *Shen Men* were also included. Infrared heat was additionally applied to the woman's feet. The patient continued this treatment for six and a half months during her pregnancy as a prevention against miscarriage.

At one point in her pregnancy, the patient caught a cold. Therefore, I prescribed *Sang Ju Fang* (Morus & Chrysanthemum Formula), *i.e.*, *Sang Ye* (Folium Mori Albi), *Ju Hua* (Flos Chrysanthemi Morifolii), *Jie Geng* (Radix Platycodi Grandiflori), *Lian Qiao* (Fructus Forsythiae Suspensae), *Lu Gen* (Rhizoma Phragmitis Communis), *Bo He* (Herba Menthae Haplocalycis), *Jing Jie Sui* (Herba Seu Flos Schizonepetae Tenuifoliae), *Xing Ren* (Semen Pruni Armeniacae), *Chen Pi* (Pericarpium Citri Reticulatae), and *Gan Cao* (Radix Glycyrrhizae Uralanesis). At another point during her pregnancy, the patient experienced severe nausea and vomiting, lower abdominal pain, and constipation which caused her to visit a hospital emergency room. For treatment, I prescribed *Liu Jun Zi Fang* (Six Gentlemen Formula) for the nausea. Modifications included a large quantity of added *Bai Shao* (Radix Albus Paeoniae Lactiflorae) to eliminate lower abdominal cramping, and *Sheng Jiang* (uncooked Rhizoma Zingiberis Officinalis) to harmonize the middle and stop nausea. *Gou Qi Zi* (Fructus Lycii Chinensis) was added to nourish the blood and promote fetal development, while crushed *Xing Ren* (Semen Pruni Armeniacae) was added to moisten the intestines and free the flow of the stools. The woman eventually gave birth to a healthy boy.

Case history 7: Ovarian cysts & IVF

The combination of Chinese medicinal formulas and acupuncture provides the most effective treatment for infertility and IVF, although I have found the Chinese herbs to be especially important in this process. However, some patients refuse herbal medicines. In that case, I treat these patients solely with acupuncture, and using acupuncture alone often brings excellent results. Nevertheless, patients receiving at least 2-3 months of support with Chinese medicinals and acupuncture obtain the best results. The following case illustrates the power of providing Chinese medicinal formulas in the treatment of infertility and the use of IVF.

One 41 year-old patient began treatment without the use of herbs when she came into the clinic. She had struggled with infertility for many years due to ovarian cysts. She had two failed IVF cycles prior to treatment with Chinese medicine. Both cycles produced very few follicles. For example, her second IVF produced only three follicles.

The patient began treatment with Chinese medicine just after starting oral contraceptive pills for her third IVF cycle. The patient chose acupuncture without herbs and was treated only a few weeks before the third IVF transfer took place. She produced only one follicle and the third cycle failed. Then the patient went on a Chinese medicinal prescription, along with acupuncture, until her fourth IVF. The fourth IVF produced nine follicles and six eggs, all of which became viable embryos for transfer. Three embryos were successfully transferred, and the patient became pregnant.

This patient's Chinese medical pattern discrimination was spleen-kidney qi and blood vacuity with liver depression qi stagnation and phlegm dampness. Signs and symptoms included fatigue and irritability with a 25 day menstrual cycle and only very light flow. Her tongue was pale with teeth-marks on its edges and white fur, while her pulse was slippery and weak in the cubit positions.

While taking oral contraceptive pills for the fourth IVF, the patient was placed on *Huo Jing Zhong Zi Fang* (Quicken the Essence & Plant the Seed Formula), *i.e.*, *Dang Gui* (Radix Angelicae Sinensis), *Chai Hu*

(Radix Bupleuri), *Bai Shao* (Radix Albus Paeoniae Lactiflorae), *Bai Zhu* (Rhizoma Atractylodis Macrocephalae), *Fu Ling* (Sclerotium Poriae Cocos), *Gan Cao* (Radix Glycyrrhizae Uralanesis), *Zhi Ke* (Fructus Citri Aurantii), and *Dan Shen* (Radix Salviae Miltiorrhize), to rectify the qi and nourish the blood. To further fortify the spleen and supplement the qi, *Dang Shen* (Radix Codonopsitis Pilosulae) was added. *Suan Zao Ren* (Semen Zizyphi Spinosae) was included to quiet the spirit, and *Dan Pi* (Cortex Radicis Moutan) was used to clear heat and quicken the blood in order to reduce anxiety and prepare for menstruation. *Gou Qi Zi* (Fructus Lycii Chinensis) was included to supplement the kidneys and nourish the blood. Acupuncture during this time included the base prescription *Zu San Li* (St 36), *San Yin Jiao* (Sp 6), *Tai Xi* (Ki 3), *Tai Chong* (Liv 3), *He Gu* (LI 4), and *Yin Tang* (M-HN-3). Then *Xue Hai* (Sp 10) was added to quicken the blood, and *Zi Gong Xue* (M-CA-18) was added to increase lower abdominal circulation and improve ovarian function. Ear points Kidney, Spleen, and *Shen Men* were added to strengthen the three main viscera responsible for reproduction—the kidneys, spleen, and liver.

When menstruating after the patient discontinued the oral contraceptive pills, she went on *Jing Qian Fang* (Menstruation-smoothing Formula), *i.e.*, *Dang Gui* (Radix Angelicae Sinensis), *Bai Shao* (Radix Albus Paeoniae Lactiflorae), *Shu Di Huang* (cooked Radix Rehmanniae Glutinosae), *Chuan Xiong* (Radix Ligustici Wallichii), *Niu Xi* (Radix Achyranthis Bidentatae), *Dan Shen* (Radix Salviae Miltiorrhizae), *Xiang Fu* (Rhizoma Cyperi Rotundi), and *Gou Qi Zi* (Fructus Lycii Chinensis), to quicken the blood. *Gui Zhi* (Ramulus Cinnamomi Cassiae) was added to warm the uterus and promote circulation. The formula was also modified with *Dang Shen* (Radix Codonopsitis Pilosulae) to fortify the spleen and supplement the qi and *Ba Ji Tian* (Radix Morindae Officinalis) to supplement the kidneys and invigorate yang. The acupuncture base prescription was the same as above plus *Xue Hai* (Sp 10), *Guan Yuan* (CV 4), and *Qi Hai* (CV 6). *Guan Yuan* and *Qi Hai* stimulate the thoroughfare vessel and increase circulation in the uterus, while *Xue Hai* moves the blood and invigorates circulation. Ear points Kidney, Spleen, and *Shen Men* were alsoincluded, as well as infrared heat.

At the start of hormonal stimulation, *Ding Jing Fang* (Stabilize the

Menses Formula), *i.e.*, *Dang Gui* (Radix Angelicae Sinensis), *Bai Shao* (Radix Albus Paeoniae Lactiflorae), *Chai Hu* (Radix Bupleuri), *Fu Ling* (Sclerotium Poriae Cocos), *Shan Yao* (Radix Dioscoreae Oppositae), *Dang Shen* (Radix Codonopsitis Pilosulae), *Ba Ji Tian* (Radix Morindae Officinalis), and mix-fried *Gan Cao* (Radix Glycyrrhizae Uralanesis), was prescribed with the addition of *Chen Pi* (Pericarpium Citri Reticulatae) to rectify the qi. *Shan Zhu Yu* (Fructus Corni Officinalis) was added to further supplement the kidneys, *Bai Zhu* (Rhizoma Atractylodis Macrocephalae) was added to further supplement the spleen, *Gou Qi Zi* (Fructus Lycii Chinensis) was added to further nourish the blood, and *Yin Yang Huo* (Herba Epimedii) was added to further invigorate yang. Acupuncture included the same base prescription as above plus *Bai Hui* (GV 20) and *Zi Gong Xue* (M-CA-18) to stimulate FSH production by the pituitary gland. Ear points Kidney, Spleen, and *Shen Men* were also used as was infrared heat.

During the transfer of embryos, both the day prior to as well as the morning of transfer, the patient took dosages of *Xiao Yao Fang* (Rambling Formula), *i.e.*, *Dang Gui* (Radix Angelicae Sinensis), *Chai Hu* (Radix Bupleuri), *Bai Shao* (Radix Albus Paeoniae Lactiflorae), *Bai Zhu* (Rhizoma Atractylodis Macrocephalae), *Fu Ling* (Sclerotium Poriae Cocos), and *Gan Cao* (Radix Glycyrrhizae Uralanesis), to supplement and rectify the qi, nourish the blood and prepare the uterus and cervix for transfer. *Zhi Ke* (Fructus Citri Aurantii) was added to harmonize the qi and loosen the cervix, thus facilitating ease of transfer into the uterus. *Dan Shen* (Radix Salviae Miltiorrhizae) was added to clear heat and quiet the spirit. *Suan Zao Ren* (Semen Zizyphi Spinosae) was also added to further quiet the spirit. *Gou Qi Zi* (Fructus Lycii Chinensis) was added to nourish the blood and supplement the kidneys. Acupuncture was again the same basic prescription, this time with *Bai Hui* (GV 20) to upbear the qi and hold the embryos and *Zi Hu-Bao Men* (Ki 13) to relax and increase the blood flow to the uterus, thereby encouraging implantation. The ear point combination of Kidney, Spleen, and *Shen Men* was included to supplement the spleen and kidneys, thereby promoting the nourishment of the uterus by strengthening the former and latter heaven roots of qi and blood engenderment and transformation. Infrared heat was also used on the patient's lower abdomen.

After transfer of the embryos, the patient continued with the base formula *Xiao Yao Fang* (Rambling Formula) modified by the addition of *Dang Shen* (Radix Codonopsitis Pilosulae), *Shan Zhu Yu* (Fructus Corni Officinalis), and *Tu Si Zi* (Semen Cuscutae Chinensis) to invigorate yang and foster the essence, thereby securing the fetus. *Suan Zao Ren* (Semen Zizyphi Spinosae) was also added to quiet the woman's spirit. Acupuncture after transfer focused on relaxing the uterus and preventing uterine contractions. This was accomplished by needling *Zu San Li* (St 36), *Bai Hui* (GV 20), *Yin Tang* (M-HN-3), and *Si Shen Cong* (M-HN-1) and ear points Kidney, Spleen, and *Shen Men* plus infrared heat on her abdomen.

Once pregnant, the patient was put on *An Tai Fang* (Safety Fetus Formula), *i.e.*, *Sang Ji Sheng* (Ramulus Sangjisheng), *Xu Duan* (Radix Dipsaci Asteri), *Tu Si Zi* (Semen Cuscutae Chinensis), *Gou Qi Zi* (Fructus Lycii Chinensis), *Shan Zhu Yu* (Fructus Corni Officinalis), *Dang Shen* (Radix Codonopsitis Pilosulae), *Bai Shao* (Radix Albus Paeoniae Lactiflorae), and *Bai Zhu* (Rhizoma Atractylodis Macrocephalae), to prevent miscarriage. The formula was modified with *E Jiao* (Gelatinum Corii Asini) to nourish the blood and stop bleeding and *Huang Qi* (Radix Astragali Membranacei) to supplement the qi and secure the fetus. Only *Bai Hui* (GV 20), *Yin Tang* (M-HN-3), and ear points Kidney, Spleen, and *Shen Men* were used, plus infrared heat on her feet to stimulate *Da Dun* (Liv 1) and *Yin Bai* (Sp 1) to prevent miscarriage.

The outcome was one healthy girl who is two years old now.

Case history 8: Irregular menstruation, low sperm count & IVF

I treated one married couple in which the wife had irregular menstruation and the husband had a low sperm count as well as weak motility. The female was 39 years old and the male was 42 years of age. The couple had two unsuccessful IVFs prior to treatment with acupuncture and Chinese medicinals. The first IVF produced 11 follicles, eight eggs, and four embryos, only one of which divided to eight cells. The patient became pregnant with this cycle. However, she miscarried early in the first trimester. In the second IVF, four eggs and only one embryo were produced. The patient did not become pregnant. In contrast, the third IVF, after utilizing acupuncture and Chinese medicinals, produced eight follicles and five high quality embryos. The treatments with Chinese medicine addressed both the husband and wife's fertility issues and improved their chances in the use of IVF. Their third IVF was successful, and today they have a two year-old baby girl.

The female patient's Chinese medical pattern discrimination was kidney and blood vacuity with qi stagnation and blood stasis. Her menstrual cycles were long and irregular, varying widely, though flowing an average of 5-6 weeks apart. Therefore, the first step was to regulate the wife's menstruation. To regulate her cycle, she was treated with *Ding Jing Fang* (Stabilize the Menses Formula) to quicken the blood and balance her hormones. This formula was modified with the addition of *Dan Shen* (Radix Salviae Miltiorrhizae) or, alternatively, *Niu Xi* (Radix Achyranthis Bidentatae) to quicken the blood. Several blood-supplementing medicinals were also added. These included *Gou Qi Zi* (Fructus Lycii Chinensis), *Huang Jing* (Rhizoma Polygonati), and *Ji Xue Teng* (Radix Et Caulis Spatholobi). For qi depression, *Xiang Fu* (Rhizoma Cyperi Rotundi), *Zhi Ke* (Fructus Citri Aurantii), and/or *Chen Pi* (Pericarpium Citri Reticulatae) were used to course the liver and move the qi. Acupuncture points included *Bai Hui* (GV 20), *Yin Tang* (M-HN-3), *Zu San Li* (St 36), *Tai Xi* (Ki 3), *San Yin Jiao* (Sp 6), *He Gu* (LI 4), and *Zi Hu-Ban Men* (Ki 13). This protocol regulated her menstrual cycles in three months and reduced her FSH level from four to two.

During the preparation for IVF, when the patient began the oral contraceptive pills, she was started on *Huo Jing Zhong Zi Fang* (Quicken the Essence & Plant the Seed Formula), *i.e.*, *Dang Gui* (Radix Angelicae Sinensis), *Chai Hu* (Radix Bupleuri), *Bai Shao* (Radix Albus Paeoniae Lactiflorae), *Bai Zhu* (Rhizoma Atractylodis Macrocephalae), *Fu Ling* (Sclerotium Poriae Cocos), *Gan Cao* (Radix Glycyrrhizae Uralanesis), *Zhi Ke* (Fructus Citri Aurantii), and *Dan Shen* (Radix Salviae Miltiorrhize), with *Gou Qi Zi* (Fructus Lycii Chinensis) and *Suan Zao Ren* (Semen Zizyphi Spinosae) as modifiers to regulate her hormones. Once the hormone injections began (this client took Gonal-F and Repronex), *Ding Jing Fang* (Stabilize the Menses Formula) was prescribed in order to produce more follicles and increase her uterine lining. *Sha Yuan Zi* (Semen Astragali Complanati) and *Huang Qi* (Radix Astragali Membranacei) were added as modifications. *Huo Jing Zhong Zi Fang* (Quicken the Essence & Plant the Seed Formula) was taken the night before as well as on the morning of the transfer, and once again *Gou Qi Zi* (Fructus Lycii Chinensis) was added to nourish the blood and *Suan Zao Ren* (Semen Zizyphi Spinosae) was added to quiet the spirit.

After transfer, *Xiao Yao Fang* (Rambling Formula) was prescribed to rectify the qi, nourish the blood, and relax the patient. *Suan Zao Ren* (Semen Zizyphi Spinosae) was added again along with *Tu Si Zi* (Semen Cuscutae Chinensis), *Dang Shen* (Radix Codonopsitis Pilosulae), *Chen Pi* (Pericarpium Citri Reticulatae), and *Shan Zhu Yu* (Fructus Corni Officinalis) to further supplement the qi and fill the essence.

Once pregnant, *An Tai Fang* (Safety Fetus Formula), *i.e.*, *Sang Ji Sheng* (Ramulus Sangjisheng), *Xu Duan* (Radix Dipsaci Asteri), *Tu Si Zi* (Semen Cuscutae Chinensis), *Gou Qi Zi* (Fructus Lycii Chinensis), *Shan Zhu Yu* (Fructus Corni Officinalis), *Dang Shen* (Radix Codonopsitis Pilosulae), *Bai Shao* (Radix Albus Paeoniae Lactiflorae), and *Bai Zhu* (Rhizoma Atractylodis Macrocephalae), was prescribed, to which *Huang Qi* (Radix Astragali Membranacei) was added to further boost the qi. At this point, acupuncture points were limited to *Bai Hui* (GV 20), *Yin Tang* (M-HN-3), and *Si Shen Cong* (M-HN-1) in order to protect a possible pregnancy. At six weeks of pregnancy, the client experienced vaginal spotting. In order to prevent miscarriage, *An Tai Fang* was modified with the addition of *Ai Ye* (Folium Artemisiae Argyi) and *E Jiao* (Gelatinum Corii Asini) to nourish and stop bleeding.

The husband had been diagnosed with having a varicocele and had completed surgical treatment several years earlier. However, this surgery did not improve the husband's condition. Laboratory analysis of the husband's sperm reported a total count of 4.4 m/ml and motility at 47%. The second step, therefore, was to increase the husband's sperm count and improve its quality. To increase sperm count and improve motility, *Huo Jing Zhong Zi Fang* (Quicken the Essence & Plant the Seed Formula), *i.e., Dang Gui* (Radix Angelicae Sinensis), *Chai Hu* (Radix Bupleuri), *Bai Shao* (Radix Albus Paeoniae Lactiflorae), *Bai Zhu* (Rhizoma Atractylodis Macrocephalae), *Fu Ling* (Sclerotium Poriae Cocos), *Gan Cao* (Radix Glycyrrhizae Uralanesis), *Zhi Ke* (Fructus Citri Aurantii), and *Dan Shen* (Radix Salviae Miltiorrhize), was prescribed with the addition of *Gui Zhi* (Ramulus Cinnamomi Cassiae) to free the flow and increase the circulation in the channels. To supplement the kidneys, enrich yin, and foster the essence, thereby improving the volume and quality of sperm, *Shan Zhu Yu* (Fructus Corni Officinalis) and *Shu Di Huang* (cooked Radix Rehmanniae Glutinosae) were added. In order to specifically improve sperm motility, *Huang Qi* (Radix Astragali Membranacei) and *Dang Shen* (Radix Codonopsitis Pilosulae) were added to supplement the qi, while *Ba Ji Tian* (Radix Morindae Officinalis) and *Rou Gui* (Cortex Cinnamomi Cassiae) were added to warm yang. Strengthening the sperm and increasing the total count improved the opportunity for conception. A greater number of viable embryos were produced, which reduced the risk of miscarriage and facilitated a successful implantation. The husband's acupuncture prescription included *Zu San Li* (St 36), *San Yin Jiao* (Sp 6), *Xue Hai* (Sp 10), *Tai Xi* (Ki 3), *Tai Chong* (Liv 3), *He Gu* (LI 4), *Qi Hai* (CV 6), *Bai Hui* (GV 20), and ear points Kidney, Spleen, and Liver.

Case history 9: Immune deficiency & IVF

A 38 year-old woman came for treatment with a history of infertility related to immunological incompatibility. Immunological examination revealed an antagonism between the husband's sperm and the wife's eggs. DQα testing revealed her DQα to be 1.22, and her husband's DQα to be 1.1. This determined whether or not the couple was so similar that the female's immune system would not produce protective antibodies to protect the fetus, because her body would not recognize the cells arising from her partner as foreign. Autoimmune phenomena, such as antiphospholipid antibodies and natural killer cell activity, are exacerbated when the mother and fetus share the same DQα or DQβ genotypes. Normal NKA (natural killer cell assay) is 2-12. The NKA results for this patient was positive at a level of 18.6.

Western medical treatment for antibody antagonism of this kind is limited and experimental. This patient was prescribed metformin (Glucophage), a medicine which has been shown to improve immune function for patients with diabetes mellitus. However, metformin has not been proven for use in treating antibody antagonism such as in this case. Many Western doctors do not agree with the use of this drug other than to treat diabetes. The patient simultaneously took Chinese medicinal prescriptions with the metformin.

The patient had a history of painful menstrual periods and PMS. She had two miscarriages in the year and a half prior to treatment with acupuncture and Chinese medicinals. Before the miscarriages, her menstrual cycles were 28-30 days apart. After the miscarriages, however, she began menstruating 38-40 days apart. She complained of frequent nightmares, frequent urination, thirst, and dry skin. She also experienced loose stools alternating with constipation. The patient was emotionally depressed. Her tongue was pale with a red tip and white fur. Her pulse was weak in both cubit positions and slippery.

Based on the above signs and symptoms, I believed the patient's Chinese medical pattern discrimination was spleen-kidney dual vacuity, and my treatment focused on strengthening the patient's immune system. This was done by first moving and quickening the qi and blood to reduce the old, antagonistic antibodies, which are considered pathogenic in Chinese medicine, since they obstruct the patient's reproductive function. Then the patient's immune system was boosted by fortifying the spleen's function of engendering and transforming new qi and blood, nourishing kidney yin and invigorating kidney yang.

Prior to her menstrual cycle, the patient took *Xiao Yao Fang* (Rambling Formula), *i.e.*, *Dang Gui* (Radix Angelicae Sinensis), *Chai Hu* (Radix Bupleuri), *Bai Shao* (Radix Albus Paeoniae Lactiflorae), *Bai Zhu* (Rhizoma Atractylodis Macrocephalae), *Fu Ling* (Sclerotium Poriae Cocos), and *Gan Cao* (Radix Glycyrrhizae Uralanesis), plus *Zhi Ke* (Fructus Citri Aurantii) to rectify the qi and *Dan Shen* (Radix Salviae Miltiorrhizae) to quicken the blood, clear heat, and quiet the patient's spirit. *Mu Dan Pi* (Cortex Radicis Moutan) was also added to quicken the blood and transform stasis. *Bai Zi Ren* (Semen Biotae Orientalis) was added to nourish heart blood and *Suan Zao Ren* (Semen Zizyphi Spinosae) was added to nourish heart and liver blood. Therefore, both these medicinals quiet the spirit. *Dang Shen* (Radix Codonopsitis Pilosulae) was added to fortify the spleen and thereby promote the engenderment and transformation of qi and blood. Acupuncture before her menstrual period consisted of *Zu San Li* (St 36), *San Yin Jiao* (Sp 6), *Tai Xi* (Ki 3), *Tai Chong* (Liv 3), *He Gu* (LI 4), *Yin Tang* (M-HN-3), *Zi Gong Xue* (M-CA-18), *Xue Hai* (Sp 10), and ear points Kidney, Spleen, and *Shen Men*.

During her menstrual period, she was placed on *Yang Jing Fang* (Nourish the Menses Formula), *i.e.*, *Dang Gui* (Radix Angelicae Sinensis), *Bai Shao* (Radix Albus Paeoniae Lactiflorae), *Shan Zhu Yu* (Fructus Corni Officinalis), *Shu Di Huang* (cooked Radix Rehmanniae Glutinosae), *Shan Yao* (Radix Dioscoreae Oppositae), *He Shou Wu* (Radix Polygoni Multiflori), *Gou Qi Zi* (Fructus Lycii Chinensis), and *Tu Si Zi* (Semen Cuscutae Chinensis), to nourish the blood. *Dan Shen* (Radix Salviae Miltiorrhizae) was added to quicken the blood, while *Xiang Fu* (Rhizoma Cyperi Rotundi) was added to move the qi, thereby promoting menstruation to flow smoothly. *Suan Zao Ren* (Semen Zizyphi Spinosae) was also added to quiet the spirit. Acupuncture was the same base prescription as above with the addition of *Guan Yuan* (CV 4), *Qi Hai* (CV 6), and ear point Liver.

After her menstrual cycle was completed, the patient began taking

Yang Jing Fang (Nourish the Menses Formula) again to continue nourishing the blood. However, now *Nu Zhen Zi* (Fructus Ligustri Lucidi)
was added to clear heat and enrich yin, while *Suan Zao Ren* (Semen
Zizyphi Spinosae) was added to nourish the blood and quiet the spirit. *Zhi Ke* (Fructus Citri Aurantii) was used to rectify the qi, and *Dan
Shen* (Radix Salviae Miltiorrhizae) was added to quicken and nourish
the blood. This latter medicinal is especially good at moving "bad
cells" out while building new, good cells. The single medicinal *Dan
Shen* is considered to be equal in function to the entire formula *Si Wu
Tang* (Four Materials Decoction), a classic Chinese prescription for the
nourishment and quickening of the blood. However, it should be noted
that moving the qi and quickening the blood is not the usual protocol
to use after a woman's menstrual cycle, when treatment normally
would focus on supplementation of the blood lost during menstruation. The purpose of continuing to move the qi and quicken the blood
in this case was to move out the poor qi and blood and replace it with
new. This is done to strengthen the immune system. The patient's
acupuncture treatment after menstruation also focused on moving the
qi and quickening the blood with the same base prescription of points
plus *Bai Hui* (GV 20) to stimulate immune responsiveness.

After three months of treatment, the patient was retested for antibody
levels, and her tests came back normal. Her FSH levels were also down
to a level of four. Therefore, in preparation for IVF, she was placed on
Huo Jing Zhong Zi Fang (Quicken the Essence & Plant the Seed
Formula), *i.e.*, *Dang Gui* (Radix Angelicae Sinensis), *Chai Hu* (Radix
Bupleuri), *Bai Shao* (Radix Albus Paeoniae Lactiflorae), *Bai Zhu*
(Rhizoma Atractylodis Macrocephalae), *Fu Ling* (Sclerotium Poriae
Cocos), *Gan Cao* (Radix Glycyrrhizae Uralanesis), *Zhi Ke* (Fructus
Citri Aurantii), and *Dan Shen* (Radix Salviae Miltiorrhize), while taking oral contraceptive pills to regulate ovarian responsiveness and pre-
pare for follicular development. *Tian Ma* (Rhizoma Gastrodiae Elatae)
was added to this prescription to treat the patient's current complaint
of headaches, while *Suan Zao Ren* (Semen Zizyphi Spinosae) was given
to quiet the patient's emotions and nourish the blood.

Once she stopped taking the oral contraceptives and her menstrual cycle was completed, she was placed on *Jing Qian Fang*
(Menstruation-smoothing Formula), *i.e.*, *Dang Gui* (Radix Angelicae

Sinensis), *Bai Shao* (Radix Albus Paeoniae Lactiflorae), *Shu Di Huang* (cooked Radix Rehmanniae Glutinosae), *Chuan Xiong* (Radix Ligustici Wallichii), *Niu Xi* (Radix Achyranthis Bidentatae), *Dan Shen* (Radix Salviae Miltiorrhizae), *Xiang Fu* (Rhizoma Cyperi Rotundi), and *Gou Qi Zi* (Fructus Lycii Chinensis), plus *Mu Dan Pi* (Cortex Radicis Moutan) to more strongly quicken the blood and dispel stasis. Blood-moving herbs regulate the reproductive hormones and are useful at this stage of preparation for IVF. *Zhi Ke* (Fructus Citri Aurantii) was added to further rectify the qi and aid in digestion of *Shu Di Huang*. Acupuncture at this time was the same, with the addition of *Xue Hai* (Sp 10) to quicken the blood, and *Guan Yuan* (CV 4) and *Qi Hai* (CV 6) to stimulate the controlling vessel and uterus as well as ovarian function.

While the patient took Fertinex 4 and Repronex for follicular development, I placed her on *Xiao Yao Fang* (Rambling Formula) for three days, then *Ding Jing Fang* (Stabilize the Menses Formula), *i.e., Dang Gui* (Radix Angelicae Sinensis), *Bai Shao* (Radix Albus Paeoniae Lactiflorae), *Chai Hu* (Radix Bupleuri), *Fu Ling* (Sclerotium Poriae Cocos), *Shan Yao* (Radix Dioscoreae Oppositae), *Dang Shen* (Radix Codonopsitis Pilosulae), *Ba Ji Tian* (Radix Morindae Officinalis), *Tu Si Zi* (Semen Cuscutae Chinensis), *Shu Di Huang* (cooked Radix Rehmanniae Glutinosae), and mix-fried *Gan Cao* (Radix Glycyrrhizae Uralanesis) for five days, and, after that, on *Yang Jing Zhong Zi Fang* (Nourish the Menses & Plant the Seed Formula), *i.e., Huang Jing* (Rhizoma Polygonati), *Shu Di Huang* (cooked Radix Rehmanniae Glutinosae), *Shan Zhu Yu* (Fructus Corni Officinalis), *Tu Si Zi* (Semen Cuscutae Chinensis), *Gou Qi Zi* (Fructus Lycii Chinensis), *Shan Yao* (Radix Dioscoreae Oppositae), *Dan Shen* (Radix Salviae Miltiorrhizae), and *Bai Shao* (Radix Albus Paeoniae Lactiflorae) for another five days.

There were 17 follicles, 15 eggs, and 12 embryos eventually produced from this IVF cycle. Five of the embryos were transferred, all of which had eight cells, and seven embryos were frozen for future use. After transfer, the patient was placed on *Yang Jing Fang* (Nourish the Menses Formula) again, modified with the addition of *Mai Men Dong* (Tuber Ophiopogonis Japonici) and *Wu Wei Zi* (Fructus Schisandrae Chinensis) to enrich yin and engender fluids, *Dang Shen* (Radix

Codonopsitis Pilosulae) to fortify the spleen and supplement the qi, and *Bai Zi Ren* (Semen Biotae Orientalis) to nourish heart blood and free the flow of the stools in order to help with constipation. Acupuncture included the same base prescription of points plus *Bai Hui* (GV 20) to upbear yang and hold the embryos, *Yin Tang* (M-HN-3) to quiet the spirit, and ear points Kidney, Spleen, and *Shen Men*. Infrared heat was also applied to her feet to mildly prevent bleeding. Unfortunately, the attempt failed and the patient did not become pregnant.

The next month, the remaining embryos were transferred and the patient did become pregnant! She was placed on *An Tai Fang* (Safety Fetus Formula), *i.e.*, *Sang Ji Sheng* (Ramulus Sangjisheng), *Xu Duan* (Radix Dipsaci Asteri), *Tu Si Zi* (Semen Cuscutae Chinensis), *Gou Qi Zi* (Fructus Lycii Chinensis), *Shan Zhu Yu* (Fructus Corni Officinalis), *Dang Shen* (Radix Codonopsitis Pilosulae), *Bai Shao* (Radix Albus Paeoniae Lactiflorae), and *Bai Zhu* (Rhizoma Atractylodis Macrocephalae), to quiet the fetus and prevent miscarriage. *Han Lian Cao* (Herba Ecliptae Prostratae) was added to stop bleeding, *Suan Zao Ren* (Semen Zizyphi Spinosae) was added to quiet the spirit and nourish the blood, and *Mai Men Dong* (Tuber Ophiopogonis Japonici) was added to supplement the kidneys and nourish yin. An extra large dosage of *Bai Shao* (Radix Albus Paeoniae Lactiflorae) was added to prevent uterine spasm and miscarriage, and *Chen Pi* (Pericarpium Citri Reticulatae) was included for nausea in early pregnancy. Acupuncture when pregnant was limited to *Bai Hui* (GV 20), *Yin Tang* (M-HN-3), and ear points Kidney, Spleen, and *Shen Men*. Infrared heat was applied to her feet.

For a cold caught at 12 weeks of pregnancy, the patient was placed on *Sang Ju Fang* (Morus & Chrysanthemum Formula), *i.e.*, *Sang Ye* (Folium Mori Albi), *Ju Hua* (Flos Chrysanthemi Morifolii), *Jie Geng* (Radix Platycodi Grandiflori), *Lian Qiao* (Fructus Forsythiae Suspensae), *Lu Gen* (Rhizoma Phragmitis Communis), *Bo He* (Herba Menthae Haplocalycis), *Jing Jie Sui* (Herba Seu Flos Schizonepetae Tenuifoliae), *Xing Ren* (Semen Pruni Armeniacae), *Chen Pi* (Pericarpium Citri Reticulatae), and *Gan Cao* (Radix Glycyrrhizae Uralanesis), for four days with *Ban Xia* (Rhizoma Pinelliae Ternatae) and *Huang Qin* (Radix Scutellariae Baicalensis) to clear heat, eliminate dampness, and transform phlegm congestion due to her cold. Then she was given *Liu Jun Zi Fang* (Six Gentlemen Formula), *i.e.*, *Dang Shen* (Radix Codonopsitis Pilosulae), *Fu Ling* (Sclerotium Poriae Cocos), *Bai Zhu* (Rhizoma Atractylodis Macrocephalae), *Ban Xia* (Rhizoma Pinelliae Ternatae), *Chen Pi* (Pericarpium Citri Reticulatae), and *Gan Cao* (Radix Glycyrrhizae Uralanesis), for another three days to reduce nausea and address some of the cold symptoms. *Liu Jun Zi Fang* was modified with the addition of *Xing Ren* (Semen Pruni Armeniacae) to regulate and rectify the lung qi, *Jie Geng* (Radix Platycodi Grandiflori) to diffuse the lungs and transform phlegm, and *Huang Qin* (Radix Scutellariae Baicalensis) to clear heat and eliminate dampness from the upper burner.

Using a combination of acupuncture and Chinese medicinals both before and during her pregnancy, this woman carried to full term and eventually gave birth to a healthy baby boy who is five months old now.

Case history 10: Acupuncture only & IVF

As mentioned above, a percentage of my patients choose not to use herbal prescriptions as part of their treatment. Acupuncture alone is still very effective in treating infertility and enhancing the responsiveness during IVF. Acupuncture point prescriptions can be used to promote the circulation of the blood in the pelvic cavity and improve ovarian function as well as relax the uterus and cervix and prevent contractions and expulsion of an embryo. Acupuncture needles also stimulate the pituitary gland, increasing and balancing hormone production.

For example, a 33 year-old client I treated in 2001 now has a two year-old healthy girl conceived with the help of acupuncture only and IVF. Her first IVF attempt, prior to using acupuncture, failed. She began acupuncture treatments at the start of her second IVF cycle and became pregnant. She produced 21 eggs and 16 embryos during that cycle.

This patient's Western medical diagnosis was infertility, while her Chinese medical pattern discrimination was kidney and blood vacuity with liver depression qi stagnation. Her symptoms were anxiety and restless sleep, thirst and occasional aching in her joints. Her tongue was pale and slightly dusky with a red tip and white fur, while her pulse was slippery and bowstring.

I started treatment on this woman with acupuncture at the start of her second IVF cycle, right when she began taking oral contraceptive pills. Acupuncture points used were *Zu San Li* (St 36), *San Yin Jiao* (Sp 6), *Xue Hai* (Sp 10), *Tai Xi* (Ki 3), *Tai Chong* (Liv 3), *He Gu* (LI 4), *Yin Tang* (M-HN-3), and *Zi Gong Xue* (M-CA-18). At this point in the treatment, this prescription's purpose was to stimulate uterine function and prepare the uterus to respond more effectively to the Western drugs. *Zi Gong Xue* helped circulate the blood around the ovaries and increased ovarian function. This point is located directly above the ovaries. *Xue Hai* quickens the blood, *San Yin Jiao* stimulates all three yin channels which connect with the uterus, and *Tai Chong* courses the liver and rectifies the qi.

Once her menstrual period began after taking oral contraceptives, the focus of treatment was altered by removing *Zi Gong Xue* and adding *Zhong Ji* (CV 3) and *Qi Hai* (CV 6). By adding *Zhong Ji* and *Qi Hai* which connect closely with the thoroughfare vessel and are located directly above the uterus, the focus is redirected to improving uterine function and facilitating the smooth flow of the menstrual cycle. *Zi Gong Xue* was removed from treatment since ovarian stimulation was not needed at this point in time.

At the start of hormonal stimulation, *Zu San Li* (St 36), *San Yin Jiao* (Sp 6), *Tai Xi* (Ki 3), *Tai Chong* (Liv 3), *He Gu* (LI 4), and ear points Kidney, Spleen, and *Shen Men* were used. *Bai Hui* (GV 20) was included to stimulate the pituitary gland to increase FSH production. Kidney and Spleen ear points also stimulate hormone production. The Spleen point also nourishes the blood and supports uterine function.

Immediately prior to the transfer of embryos, the same base prescription of points were used at the start of hormone stimulation (above) with the addition of *Zi Hu-Bao Men* (Ki 13). *Zi Hu-Bao Men* is located above the uterus and functions to relax the cervix so transfer is easier. It further supports implantation of the embryo by relaxing the uterus. *Si Shen Cong* (M-HN-1) was also added to calm the patient and relax the uterus, decreasing contractions which can have the negative effect of expulsion of the embryos. Infrared heat was applied to warm her abdomen.

After transfer of the embryos, *Tai Chong* (Liv 3), *San Yin Jiao* (Sp 6), and *He Gu* (LI 4) were not used since they stimulate uterine contractions. *Zu San Li* (St 36) was stimulated as well as *Tai Xi* (Ki 3), *Yin Tang* (M-HN-3), and ear points Kidney, Spleen, and *Shen Men*. *Bai Hui* (GV 20) was used to upbear the qi and secure the embryo, and *Si Shen Cong* (M-HN-1) was needled to calm the patient and relax the uterus.

Once I knew the patient was pregnant, acupuncture was limited to preventing miscarriage. Her prescription included ear points Kidney, Spleen, and *Shen Men*, *Bai Hui* (GV 20), *Si Shen Cong* (M-HN-1), and *Yin Tang* (M-HN-3). Infrared heat was applied to her feet to warm and stimulate *Da Dun* (Liv 1) and *Yin Bai* (Sp 1) in order to prevent miscarriage. The effect of infrared heat is similar to the use of moxibustion at these points.

Case history 11: Poor sperm analysis

Acupuncture and Chinese medicinals can assist couples in becoming pregnant when dealing with male infertility factors just as they can when dealing with female infertility issues. For example, one couple I treated came in with a Western medical diagnosis of male infertility caused by a varicocele. This led to poor sperm motility and morphology. The husband's semen analysis reported a total count of 80 m/ml, a volume of 2.5ml, a motility count of 18 m/ml, and a motility percentage of 22%. Gross morphology was very low, reported at only 4%. Normal values for each of these qualities are a total count greater than 25 m/ml and a volume of greater than 2.0 m/ml, while a normal percentage of motility is considered greater than 50%. A healthy morphology is greater than 50%.

The husband's Chinese medical pattern discrimination was kidney and blood vacuity with qi stagnation and blood stasis. His symptoms included fatigue, dizziness, stress and anxiety, poor digestion, including flatulence, abdominal distention, and occasional nausea, as well as chest oppression and pain. He caught a cold during the course of treatment. He also experienced ongoing back and knee pain and soreness and an aggravation of a rib injury. His tongue was red and dusky with white fur. His pulse was small, bowstring, and weak in both cubit positions.

Based on the above, I chose *Xiao Yao Fang* (Rambling Formula), *i.e.*, *Dang Gui* (Radix Angelicae Sinensis), *Chai Hu* (Radix Bupleuri), *Bai Shao* (Radix Albus Paeoniae Lactiflorae), *Bai Zhu* (Rhizoma Atractylodis Macrocephalae), *Fu Ling* (Sclerotium Poriae Cocos), and *Gan Cao* (Radix Glycyrrhizae Uralanesis), as this patient's base prescription. Modifications were added and/or removed as needed during the course of treatment. For improving sperm motility, *Ba Ji Tian* (Radix Morindae Officinalis), *Tu Si Zi* (Semen Cuscutae Chinensis), and *Sha Yuan Zi* (Semen Astragali Complanati) were added. *Ba Ji Tian* and *Tu Si Zi* both supplement the kidneys and invigorate yang, while *Tu Si Zi* also enriches yin. Sperm morphology can be enhanced by increasing the blood flow to the testicles. Therefore, *Dan Shen* (Radix Salviae Miltiorrhizae) was added for that purpose. To increase the sperm count and volume, *Shan Zhu Yu* (Fructus Corni Officinalis) and

Shu Di Huang (cooked Radix Rehmanniae Glutinosae) were added to nourish the blood and supplement yin. For the patient's low energy, *Huang Qi* (Radix Astragali Membranacei) and *Dang Shen* (Radix Codonopsitis Pilosulae) were added, and, to improve sleep, *Suan Zao Ren* (Semen Zizyphi Spinosae) was added. For chest oppression and pain, *Tao Ren* (Semen Pruni Persicae) or *Jie Geng* (Radix Platycodi Grandiflori) were included. *Chen Pi* (Pericarpium Citri Reticulatae) was added to improve digestion and reduce abdominal distention and flatulence. Since the patient suffered from high stress and anxiety and showed signs of heat, *Zhi Ke* (Fructus Citri Aurantii), *Zhi Zi* (Fructus Gardeniae Jasminoidis), and *Dan Pi* (Cortex Radicis Moutan) were used to course the liver and rectify the qi, clear heat and resolve depression. *Mai Men Dong* (Tuber Ophiopogonis Japonici) helped nourish heart yin and drain heart Fire so as to alleviate anxiety. *Gou Qi Zi* (Fructus Lycii Chinensis) was used to nourish the blood and help reduce the patient's dizziness, while *Ban Xia* (Rhizoma Pinelliae Ternatae) was added for nausea.

The basic acupuncture prescription I used with this patient for improving sperm quality was *Zu San Li* (St 36), *San Yin Jiao* (Sp 6), *Tai Xi* (Ki 3), *Tai Chong* (Liv 3), *He Gu* (LI 4), and *Yin Tang* (M-HN-3). Modifications over the course of treatment included the addition of *Zi Hu-Bao Men* (Ki 13) with *Guan Yuan* (CV 4) and *Qi Hai* (CV 6) for improving testicular function and sperm production. *Bai Hui* (GV 20) was used to stimulate the pituitary gland for production of FSH which stimulates the testes to produce testosterone. *Xue Hai* (Sp 10) was added to quicken the blood. *Tian Shu* (St 25) was used to regulate and improve digestion. Ear points Kidney, Spleen, and *Shen Men* were used together since they address the major viscera responsible for reproduction and fertility. The kidneys store the essence and are the root for overall growth and reproductive capability, while the spleen is responsible for latter heaven engenderment and transformation of the qi and blood. *Shen Men* quiets the spirit and promotes the smooth and easy flow of the liver qi. The liver qi controls the qi mechanism and an uninhibited qi mechanism is essential to physiological health.

The patient's on going back and knee pain were treated with Chinese medicinals added to the base prescription, *Xiao Yao Fang* (Rambling Formula). *Niu Xi* (Radix Achyranthis Bidentatae) and *Sang Ji Sheng*

(Ramulus Sangjisheng) were added to assuage impediment and relieve pain by quickening the blood and guiding the effects of the formula to the low back and knees. For the rib injury causing soreness, *Gui Zhi* (Ramulus Cinnamomi Cassiae), *Yan Hu Suo* (Rhizoma Corydalis Yanhusuo), and *San Qi* (Radix Notoginseng) were added to free the flow of the channels and relieve pain. Acupuncture points used to treat body pain were *Fei Shu* (Bl 13), *Xi Shu* (Bl 15), *Pi Shu* (Bl 20), *Shen Shu* (Bl 23), *Da Chang Shu* (Bl 25), *Wei Zhong* (Bl 40), *Cheng Shan* (Bl 57), *Kun Lun* (Bl 60), and *Tai Xi* (Ki 3). These urinary bladder channel points not only reduced his back and knee pain by local channel stimulation, they benefitted the overall condition of sperm quality due to their direct relationship with the internal organ systems. *Dan Zhong* (CV 17) and *Ri Yue* (GB 24) were used to loosen his chest and relieve rib-side pain.

To treat this patient's common cold, he was prescribed *Xiao Chai Hu Fang* (Minor Bupleurum Formula), *i.e.*, *Chai Hu* (Radix Bupleuri), *Dang Shen* (Radix Codonopsitis Pilosulae), *Da Zao* (Fructus Zizyphi Jujubae), *Ban Xia* (Rhizoma Pinelliae Ternatae), *Gan Cao* (Radix Glycyrrhizae Uralanesis), *Sheng Jiang* (uncooked Rhizoma Zingiberis Officinalis), and *Huang Qin* (Radix Scutellariae Baicalensis), modified by the addition of *Qing Hao* (Herba Artemisiae Annuae) and *Chen Pi* (Pericarpium Citri Reticulatae) for bloating and gas, *Fu Ling* (Sclerotium Poriae Cocos) to fortify his spleen, and *Xing Ren* (Semen Pruni Armeniacae) to stop cough. Acupuncture points to treat the cold symptoms included *Lie Que* (Lu 7) to downbear and depurate the lungs, *Yin Tang* (M-HN-3) to dispel wind, *Wai Guan* (TB 5) and *Qu Chi* (LI 11) to resolve the exterior, rectify the qi, and quicken the blood. *Tian Rong* (SI 17) and *Ting Hui* (GB 2) were used for ear congestion due to the cold.

After three months of treatment, the patient's wife became pregnant without the use of IVF or other interventions. Unfortunately she miscarried. Treatment continued with the husband for another two months until his wife conceived again. They now have a three month-old baby girl. (See the following case history for the wife's story.)

Case history 12: Abnormal cervix & low progesterone

A diagnosis of infertility due to scarring in the cervix and low progesterone brought a client in for treatment. The patient was also 42 years
old, an advanced maternal age according to Western medicine, and
presented with a history of abnormal Pap smears. Surgical removal of
the abnormal cells resulted in a narrowing of the cervical os due to the
formation of scar tissue. The patient was unable to become pregnant
for more than two years prior to treatment with Chinese medicine.
Complicating the patient's difficulties in becoming pregnant were her
husband's poor sperm motility and morphology which I also treated
with acupuncture and Chinese medicinals. (See the previous case history.) She and her husband had tried two IUIs with clomiphene citrate
(Clomid) before coming in for treatment with acupuncture and
Chinese medicinals. Unfortunately, both IUI procedures were painful
and difficult due to scar tissue blocking the patient's cervical os and
neither resulted in pregnancy.

The Chinese medical pattern discrimination for this patient was kidney
and blood vacuity with qi stagnation and blood stasis. The patient
reported symptoms of fatigue, frequent colds, hemorrhoids, PMS,
irregular sleep, tinnitus, and high stress. She also experienced leg pain
due to a blood clot in her left leg for which she had surgery one year
prior to her first acupuncture appointment. The patient's bowel movements and urination were both normal. Her tongue was slightly pale
with a red tip and white fur. Her pulse was slippery and slightly bowstring. It was also bilaterally weak in the cubit position. Treatment
principles for this case were to supplement the kidneys, course the liver
and resolve depression, quicken the blood and transform stasis.

Before she began her menstrual period, the patient took the base for-
mula *Xiao Yao Fang* (Rambling Formula), *i.e.*, *Dang Gui* (Radix
Angelicae Sinensis), *Chai Hu* (Radix Bupleuri), *Bai Shao* (Radix
Albus Paeoniae Lactiflorae), *Bai Zhu* (Rhizoma Atractylodis
Macrocephalae), *Fu Ling* (Sclerotium Poriae Cocos), and *Gan Cao*
(Radix Glycyrrhizae Uralanesis). This was modified with the addition
of *Dang Shen* (Radix Codonopsitis Pilosulae) to fortify the spleen and
supplement the qi, *Shu Di Huang* (cooked Radix Rehmanniae
Glutinosae) to nourish the blood, and *Chen Pi* (Pericarpium Citri

Reticulatae) to prevent stagnation due to the slimy, enriching nature of *Shu Di Huang*. *Gou Qi Zi* (Fructus Lycii Chinensis) was also included to nourish the blood and emolliate the liver, supplement the kidneys and enrich yin. Acupuncture at this time included the base prescription *Zu San Li* (St 36), *San Yin Jiao* (Sp 6), *Tai Chong* (Liv 3), *He Gu* (LI 4), *Tai Xi* (Ki 3), *Yin Tang* (M-HN-3), *Bai Hui* (GV 20), and ear points Kidney, Spleen, and *Shen Men*. Infrared heat was also applied to her low abdomen.

During menstruation, which were very light in blood flow, the patient was placed on *Huo Jing Zhong Zi Fang* (Quicken the Essence & Plant the Seed Formula), *i.e.*, *Dang Gui* (Radix Angelicae Sinensis), *Chai Hu* (Radix Bupleuri), *Bai Shao* (Radix Albus Paeoniae Lactiflorae), *Bai Zhu* (Rhizoma Atractylodis Macrocephalae), *Fu Ling* (Sclerotium Poriae Cocos), *Gan Cao* (Radix Glycyrrhizae Uralanesis), *Zhi Ke* (Fructus Citri Aurantii), and *Dan Shen* (Radix Salviae Miltiorrhize), to nourish and quicken the blood. *Shu Di Huang* (cooked Radix Rehmanniae Glutinosae) was added to further nourish the blood and foster the essence. *Niu Xi* (Radix Achyranthis Bidentatae) was added to nourish and enrich the liver and kidneys and promote a smooth flowing menstrual cycle. *Yi Mu Cao* (Herba Leonuri Heterophylli) was added alternatively to quicken the blood and also promote normal menstruation. *San Qi* (Radix Notoginseng) was added to quicken the blood and relieve pain. *Bai Ji Tian* (Radix Morindae Officinalis) was used to supplement the kidneys and invigorate yang so as to promote ovulation. This is because kidney yang is responsible for the stimulation and maturation of follicles so that ovulation can take place. The moving medicinals in this formula were included to promote the action of ovulation. *Dang Shen* (Radix Codonopsitis Pilosulae) was added to fortify the spleen and supplement the qi to strengthen its function of engendering and transforming new blood. Acupuncture during menstruation included the same base point prescription plus *Qu Quan* (Liv 8) to quicken and nourish the blood and *Yin Ling Quan* (Sp 9) and *Yang Ling Quan* (GB 34) to treat a local knee injury.

After menstruation, the patient was again placed on *Xiao Yao Fang* (Rambling Formula) modified for specific symptoms as necessary. For instance, *Huang Qi* (Radix Astragali Membranacei) was added for low energy, *Chen Pi* (Pericarpium Citri Reticulatae) was added for abdominal distention and flatulence, and *Shu Di Huang* (cooked Radix Rehmanniae Glutinosae) was added to increase the thickness of her uterine lining. The main focus at this point was to nourish blood and enrich yin to support the uterus. A thick endometrial lining is preferred to aid implantation and provide nourishment for the embryo. If there is poor blood circulation, such as with this client, ovarian function can be decreased and hormones, such as estrogen and progesterone, will not be produced in adequate amounts. Acupuncture after menstruation consisted of the basic point prescription outlined above. However, *Zi Gong Xue* (M-CA-18), was also included.

During ovulation, *Dan Shen* (Radix Salviae Miltiorrhizae) was added to increase blood circulation for egg development. *Ba Ji Tian* (Radix Morindae Officinalis) was added at ovulation for the purpose of supplementing the kidneys and invigorating yang. *Tu Si Zi* (Semen Cuscutae Chinensis) also was added not only to invigorate yang but also to boost the essence, stimulate ovarian function, and improve egg quality. *Yin Yang Huo* (Herba Epimedii) was added at times to increase sexual desire and make the uterus more responsive. (*Yin Yang Huo* can also assist in invigorating sperm motility.) *Suan Zao Ren* (Semen Zizyphi Spinosae) was an important addition to this particular patient's formula due to the fact that the patient had high stress, anxiety, and poor sleep. *Gou Qi Zi* (Fructus Lycii Chinensis) was used to stop heart palpitations and nourish the blood. *Gui Zhi* (Ramulus Cinnamomi Cassiae) was added to improve circulation in the channels to address leg pain due to blood stasis.

During pregnancy, it is important to protect the fetus. You must not move the qi too much or move it downward. Toxic medicinals must also be avoided, such as *Xi Xin* (Herba Asari Cum Radice) and *Tian Hua Fen* (Radix Trichosanthis Kirlowii). When this patient caught a cold during pregnancy, she was placed on *Sang Ju Fang* (Morus & Chrysanthemum Formula), *i.e.*, *Sang Ye* (Folium Mori Albi), *Ju Hua* (Flos Chrysanthemi Morifolii), *Jie Geng* (Radix Platycodi Grandiflori), *Lian Qiao* (Fructus Forsythiae Suspensae), *Lu Gen* (Rhizoma Phragmitis Communis), *Bo He* (Herba Menthae Haplocalycis), *Jing Jie Sui* (Herba Seu Flos Schizonepetae Tenuifoliae), *Xing Ren* (Semen Pruni Armeniacae), *Chen Pi* (Pericarpium Citri Reticulatae), and *Gan Cao* (Radix Glycyrrhizae Uralanesis). This was modified by the addition of *Ban Xia* (Rhizoma Pinelliae Ternatae) to transform phlegm and *Chen Pi* (Pericarpium Citri Reticulatae) to rectify the qi and eliminate dampness. For cough during pregnancy, I prescribed *Zhi Ke Fang* (Stop Cough Formula), *i.e., Ban Xia* (Rhizoma Pinelliae Ternatae), *Chen Pi* (Pericarpium Citri Reticulatae), *Fu Ling* (Sclerotium Poriae Cocos), *Gan Cao* (Radix Glycyrrhizae Uralanesis), *Xing Ren* (Semen Pruni Armeniacae), *Jie Geng* (Radix Platycodi Grandiflori), *Kuan Dong Hua* (Flos Tussilaginis Farfarae), and *Jing Jie Sui* (Herba Seu Flos Schizonepetae Tenuifoliae), plus *Huang Qin* (Radix Scutellariae Baicalensis) to clear heat and dry dampness and *Sheng Jiang* (uncooked Rhizoma Zingiberis Officinalis) to resolve the exterior. To alleviate the symptoms of common cold, *Qu Chi* (LI 11) and *Wai Guan* (TB 5) were used to resolve the exterior and dispel wind. Other points used at this time were *Dan Zhong (*CV 17) to loosen the chest, *Lie Que* (Lu 7) to regulate and rectify the lung qi, *Zu San Li* (St 36) and *Feng Long* (St 40) to transform phlegm, and *Bai Hui* (GV 20) to hold the fetus and prevent miscarriage.

Case history 13: Amenorrhea & infertility

Amenorrhea is yet another cause of infertility that can be successfully treated with acupuncture and Chinese medicinals. For example, I treated a 35 year-old patient who had been struggling with the absence of menstrual cycles for most of her life. In her entire life, she had had only five menstrual cycles without the use of hormone supplementation to force her cycle. From 23-33 years of age, she was on oral contraceptive pills in order to achieve menstruation. Her FSH level was reported to be 6.5. After one month of treatment with acupuncture and Chinese medicinals, the patient's menses returned with regularity and, within nine months, she was pregnant without the use of Western medical intervention for conception. The patient shared with me how amazed her Western medical practitioners were that she had been able to become pregnant without IVF.

Based on a pattern discrimination of kidney and blood vacuity, treatment was focused on establishing and maintaining a regular menstrual cycle, lowering her FSH level, and facilitating a successful pregnancy. To get pregnant, the patient ceased taking oral contraceptives for the two years prior to beginning treatment with acupuncture and Chinese medicinals. During those two years, she tried four IUIs with hormone supplementation (and achieved one pregnancy, which miscarried at 12 weeks), and two unsuccessful IVF cycles. In both of her IVF cycles, only nine eggs and four embryos were produced. This is a good example of how poorly her ovaries were functioning.

To establish a menstrual cycle, the patient was placed on *Jing Qian Fang* (Menstruation-smoothing Formula), *i.e.*, *Dang Gui* (Radix Angelicae Sinensis), *Bai Shao* (Radix Albus Paeoniae Lactiflorae), *Shu Di Huang* (cooked Radix Rehmanniae Glutinosae), *Chuan Xiong* (Radix Ligustici Wallichii), *Niu Xi* (Radix Achyranthis Bidentatae), *Dan Shen* (Radix Salviae Miltiorrhizae), *Xiang Fu* (Rhizoma Cyperi Rotundi), and *Gou Qi Zi* (Fructus Lycii Chinensis) for one week to quicken the blood and promote menstruation. This formula was modified with the addition of *Ba Ji Tian* (Radix Morindae Officinalis) to warm and invigorate kidney yang and *Dang Shen* (Radix Codonopsitis Pilosulae) to fortify the spleen and supplement the qi. The patient was also treated with acupuncture points *Zu San Li* (St 36), *San Yin Jiao*

(Sp 6), *Xue Hai* (Sp 10), *Tai Xi* (Ki 3), *Tai Chong* (Liv 3), *Guan Yuan* (CV 4), *Qi Hai* (CV 6), *Bai Hui* (GV 20), and *Yin Tang* (M-HN-3).

When her cycle did not begin, she was placed on *Ding Jing Fang* (Stabilize the Menses Formula), *i.e.*, *Dang Gui* (Radix Angelicae Sinensis), *Bai Shao* (Radix Albus Paeoniae Lactiflorae), *Chai Hu* (Radix Bupleuri), *Fu Ling* (Sclerotium Poriae Cocos), *Shan Yao* (Radix Dioscoreae Oppositae), *Dang Shen* (Radix Codonopsitis Pilosulae), *Ba Ji Tian* (Radix Morindae Officinalis), *Tu Si Zi* (Semen Cuscutae Chinensis), *Shu Di Huang* (cooked Radix Rehmanniae Glutinosae), and mix-fried *Gan Cao* (Radix Glycyrrhizae Uralanesis), for three weeks to nourish and quicken the blood. This formula was modified with the addition of *Rou Gui* (Cortex Cinnamomi Cassiae) to warm yang and promote the engenderment and transformation of qi and blood. *Yin Yang Huo* (Herba Epimedii) was also added to supplement both kidney yin and yang. The patient's cycles then became regular.

As stated above, once the woman's menses became regular, it took nine months for her to become pregnant. Once the patient had become pregnant, she was placed on *An Tai Fang* (Safety Fetus Formula), *i.e.*, *Sang Ji Sheng* (Ramulus Sangjisheng), *Xu Duan* (Radix Dipsaci Asteri), *Tu Si Zi* (Semen Cuscutae Chinensis), *Gou Qi Zi* (Fructus Lycii Chinensis), *Shan Zhu Yu* (Fructus Corni Officinalis), *Dang Shen* (Radix Codonopsitis Pilosulae), *Bai Shao* (Radix Albus Paeoniae Lactiflorae), and *Bai Zhu* (Rhizoma Atractylodis Macrocephalae), to prevent miscarriage. *Suan Zao Ren* (Semen Zizyphi Spinosae) was added to nourish and enrich yin and blood and quiet the spirit. *Huang Qi* (Radix Astragali Membranacei) was added to upbear the qi, thus helping to prevent miscarriage and supplementing the patient's qi. Acupuncture points *Bai Hui* (GV 20), *Yin Tang* (M-HN-3), and *Si Shen Cong* (M-HN-1) were included to also protect the pregnancy.

The baby was born on May 13, 2003. It was a very healthy girl, 7.8 pounds in weight.

Case history 14: Endometriosis & IVF

A 32 year-old patient presented with a history of endometriosis. In the past, she had also had a 3cm diameter ovarian cyst surgically removed. Her FSH was reported at 8.1. The patient had three prior attempts with IVF before treatment with acupuncture and Chinese medicinals, none of which had resulted in pregnancy. After being treated with Chinese medicine, the patient's fourth IVF resulted in a successful pregnancy. Fifteen embryos were produced, all of which were of much better quality than in the prior three IVF cycles. Seven of the embryos were frozen, and three were transferred. The transfer resulted in triplets! However, only twins were born since one fetus died in utero at 15 weeks of gestation.

Treatment began based on her Chinese medical pattern discrimination of kidney yin and yang vacuity with qi stagnation and blood stasis as well as her Western medical diagnosis of endometriosis leading to infertility. The patient's symptoms included high blood pressure (130/95mmHg at the initial consultation), irritability and cramping prior to menstruation, and a history of decreased hearing in both ears. Her pulses were weak in both the right and left cubit positions and were bowstring overall.

The first step in my preparing her for IVF was to treat her endometriosis. Therefore, the patient was started on *Huo Jing Zhong Zi Fang* (Quicken the Essence & Plant the Seed Formula), *i.e.*, *Dang Gui* (Radix Angelicae Sinensis), *Chai Hu* (Radix Bupleuri), *Bai Shao* (Radix Albus Paeoniae Lactiflorae), *Bai Zhu* (Rhizoma Atractylodis Macrocephalae), *Fu Ling* (Sclerotium Poriae Cocos), *Gan Cao* (Radix Glycyrrhizae Uralanesis), *Zhi Ke* (Fructus Citri Aurantii), and *Dan Shen* (Radix Salviae Miltiorrhize), and kept on this formula for several weeks. Before and during her menstrual cycle, *Yan Hu Suo* (Rhizoma Corydalis Yanhusuo) was added to quicken the blood, move the qi, and relieve pain. *Niu Xi* (Radix Achyranthis Bidentatae) was also added to quicken the blood and transform stasis, and *Suan Zao Ren* (Semen Zizyphi Spinosae) was added to quiet the spirit since the patient was anxious. Acupuncture points used before the patient's menstruation were *Zu San Li* (St 36), *San Yin Jiao* (Sp 6), *Xue Hai* (Sp 10), *Tai Xi* (Ki 3), *Tai Chong* (Liv 3), *He Gu* (LI 4), *Guan Yuan* (CV

4), *Qi Hai* (CV 6), and *Yin Tang* (M-HN-3). Infrared heat was also applied to the lower abdomen during treatment.

After her menstruation, the base prescription was modified with *Tu Si Zi* (Semen Cuscutae Chinensis) to nourish and invigorate the kidney yin and yang, *Ba Ji Tian* (Radix Morindae Officinalis) to supplement the kidneys and invigorate yang, and *Shu Di Huang* (cooked Radix Rehmanniae Glutinosae) to nourish the blood and enrich yin. The above acupuncture prescription was modified by removing *Guan Yuan* (CV 4) *Qi Hai* (CV 6), and *Xue Hai* (Sp 10) and adding *Zi Gong Xue* (M-CA-18).

Once the IVF program began, the initial formula for the patient was *Xiao Yao Fang* (Rambling Formula), *i.e., Dang Gui* (Radix Angelicae Sinensis), *Chai Hu* (Radix Bupleuri), *Bai Shao* (Radix Albus Paeoniae Lactiflorae), *Bai Zhu* (Rhizoma Atractylodis Macrocephalae), *Fu Ling* (Sclerotium Poriae Cocos), and *Gan Cao* (Radix Glycyrrhizae Uralanesis), to rectify the qi and nourish the blood. This prescription was modified with the addition of *Dang Shen* (Radix Codonopsitis Pilosulae) to supplement the qi, *Tu Si Zi* (Semen Cuscutae Chinensis) to invigorate yang and boost the essence, *Shu Di Huang* (cooked Radix Rehmanniae Glutinosae) to nourish the blood and enrich yin, and *Zhi Ke* (Fructus Citri Aurantii) to aid in the digestion of the formula. When needed, the formula was also modified with *Niu Xi* (Radix Achyranthis Bidentatae) to guide the action of the formula to the lower abdomen and to nourish and enrich the liver and kidneys as well as to promote the smooth flow of blood. *Ba Ji Tian* (Radix Morindae Officinalis) was added to supplement the kidneys and invigorate yang. Once the IVF procedure had been completed, the patient chose to discontinue the use of herbs as part of her course of treatment.

During IVF, when the patient started oral contraceptive pills, she was taken off of the above Chinese medicinals as per request by her Western M.D., and given acupuncture at *Zu San Li* (St 36), *San Yin Jiao* (Sp 6), *Xue Hai* (Sp 10), *Tai Xi* (Ki 3), *Tai Chong* (Liv 3), *He Gu* (LI 4), *Guan Yuan* (CV 4), *Qi Hai* (CV 6), *Yin Tang* (M-HN-3), and *Zi Gong Xue* (M-CA-18). Once ovarian stimulation began, the acupuncture prescription above was modified to include ear points Kidney, Spleen, and *Shen Men*.

After transfer had taken place, the patient went back on Chinese medicinals, taking *An Tai Fang* (Safety Fetus Formula), *i.e.*, *Sang Ji Sheng* (Ramulus Sangjisheng), *Xu Duan* (Radix Dipsaci Asteri), *Tu Si Zi* (Semen Cuscutae Chinensis), *Gou Qi Zi* (Fructus Lycii Chinensis), *Shan Zhu Yu* (Fructus Corni Officinalis), *Dang Shen* (Radix Codonopsitis Pilosulae), *Bai Shao* (Radix Albus Paeoniae Lactiflorae), and *Bai Zhu* (Rhizoma Atractylodis Macrocephalae), to support a possible pregnancy. This formula was modified by the addition of *Huang Qi* (Radix Astragali Membranacei) to supplement the qi and *Suan Zao Ren* (Semen Zizyphi Spinosae) to nourish and enrich yin and blood and quiet the spirit. Acupuncture points *Bai Hui* (GV 20), *Si Shen Cong* (M-HN-1), *Yin Tang* (M-HN-3), and ear points Kidney, Spleen, and *Shen Men* were used to help maintain her pregnancy. The pregnancy went to full term and the patient gave birth to twins as mentioned above.

Case history 15: High FSH & IVF

A 32 year-old patient was diagnosed as infertile due to high FSH levels. Her FSH was reported at 17. Prior to treatment with acupuncture and Chinese medicinals, she had attempted two IUI procedures. She became pregnant with both IUI procedures, but she miscarried both within 5-6 weeks of conception. High FSH is directly related to poor ovarian function. Acupuncture and Chinese medicinals along with IVF were the next steps chosen by this patient. She became pregnant during the first IVF cycle and has successfully carried the pregnancy into the third trimester.

This patient's Chinese medical pattern discrimination was kidney and blood vacuity with liver depression qi stagnation. Therefore, my treatment focused on supplementing the kidneys and nourishing the blood as well as coursing the liver and rectifying the qi. Her signs and symptoms included fatigue, headaches, and a regular menstrual cycle with normal bleeding of 5-6 days duration every 28 days. Her tongue was red, dusky, and small in size with a dry, white fur. She also had slight teeth-marks along the sides of her tongue. Her pulse was weak in both cubit positions and slippery.

The patient decided to use only acupuncture and to not take an herbal prescription prior to transfer in the IVF cycle. Acupuncture points used consisted of *Zu San Li* (St 36), *San Yin Jiao* (Sp 6), *Tai Xi* (Ki 3), *Tai Chong* (Liv 3), *He Gu* (LI 4), *Yin Tang* (M-HN-3), and *Zi Gong Xue* (M-CA-18). Infrared heat was also applied to her lower abdomen. During hormonal stimulation with Lupron and Gonal F, the same base acupuncture prescription as above was used with the inclusion of *Bai Hui* (GV 20). Six follicles, six eggs, and five embryos were produced in the cycle, and three embryos were transferred. Using the same base points plus *Zi Hu-Bao Men* (Ki 13), *Bai Hui* (GV 20), and *Si Shen Cong* (M-HN-1) helped calm the patient and relaxed her uterus to facilitate implantation. Ear points Kidney, Spleen, and *Shen Men* were included to prevent miscarriage. Infrared heat was again applied to her lower abdomen.

After the embryos were transferred, the patient began taking Chinese medicinals, starting with *Yang Tai Fang* (Nourish the Fetus Formula), *i.e.*, *Tu Si Zi* (Semen Cuscutae Chinensis), *Shu Di Huang* (cooked Radix Rehmanniae Glutinosae), *Shan Zhu Yu* (Fructus Corni Officinalis), *Shan Yao* (Radix Dioscoreae Oppositae), *Bai Shao* (Radix Albus Paeoniae Lactiflorae), *Mai Men Dong* (Tuber Ophiopogonis Japonici), *Suan Zao Ren* (Semen Zizyphi Spinosae), and *Gan Cao* (Radix Glycyrrhizae Uralanesis), to prevent miscarriage by invigorating yang and nourishing the blood. *Dang Shen* (Radix Codonopsitis Pilosulae) was added to further supplement the qi and *Wu Wei Zi* (Fructus Schisandrae Chinensis) was added to nourish yin. Acupuncture points used at this time were *Zu San Li* (St 36) to supplement the qi and nourish the blood, *Tai Xi* (Ki 3) to supplement the kidneys and nourish yin, *Bai Hui* (GV 20) to upbear the qi, and ear points Kidney, Spleen, and *Shen Men*.

An Tai Fang (Safety Fetus Formula), *i.e.*, *Sang Ji Sheng* (Ramulus Sangjisheng), *Xu Duan* (Radix Dipsaci Asteri), *Tu Si Zi* (Semen Cuscutae Chinensis), *Gou Qi Zi* (Fructus Lycii Chinensis), *Shan Zhu Yu* (Fructus Corni Officinalis), *Dang Shen* (Radix Codonopsitis Pilosulae), *Bai Shao* (Radix Albus Paeoniae Lactiflorae), and *Bai Zhu* (Rhizoma Atractylodis Macrocephalae), was prescribed once the patient became pregnant in order to nourish and enrich yin and blood and to prevent miscarriage. *Han Lian Cao* (Herba Ecliptae Prostratae) was added to stop bleeding and help prevent miscarriage. *Suan Zao Ren* (Semen Zizyphi Spinosae) was added to nourish the blood, secure and astringe, and quiet the spirit, and *Sheng Jiang* (uncooked Rhizoma Zingiberis Officinalis) was added to reduce nausea.

The patient caught a cold during this pregnancy. Therefore, I prescribed *Sang Ju Fang* (Morus & Chrysanthemum Formula), *i.e.*, *Sang Ye* (Folium Mori Albi), *Ju Hua* (Flos Chrysanthemi Morifolii), *Jie Geng* (Radix Platycodi Grandiflori), *Lian Qiao* (Fructus Forsythiae Suspensae), *Lu Gen* (Rhizoma Phragmitis Communis), *Bo He* (Herba Menthae Haplocalycis), *Jing Jie Sui* (Herba Seu Flos Schizonepetae Tenuifoliae), *Xing Ren* (Semen Pruni Armeniacae), *Chen Pi* (Pericarpium Citri Reticulatae), and *Gan Cao* (Radix Glycyrrhizae Uralanesis). Great care was taken to avoid medicinals which might be too dispersing and, thus, adversely effect the pregnancy. *Ban Xia* (Rhizoma Pinelliae Ternatae) was added to the formula to dry dampness and reduce nausea. Acupuncture included only *Bai Hui* (GV 20),

Si Shen Cong (M-HN-1), *Yin Tang* (M-HN-3), and ear points Kidney, Spleen, and *Shen Men* to prevent miscarriage. Infrared heat was applied only to her feet to mildly stimulate *Da Dun* (Liv 1) and *Yin Bai* (Sp 1) to prevent bleeding. As of this writing, the patient is eight and a half months pregnant and everything is progressing fine.

Appendix 1

Recent Research on Acupuncture & IVF

In an article published by W. Paulus, M. Zhang, I. El-Danasouri, E. Strehler and K. Sterzik titled, "Influence of Acupuncture on the Pregnancy Rate in Patients Who Undergo Assisted Reproduction Therapy," appearing in the April 2002 issue of *Fertility and Sterility*, German researchers announced that they had increased the success rate by nearly 50% in women undergoing *in vitro* fertilization. The researchers, led by Dr. Wolfgang E. Paulus and colleagues at the Christian-Lauritzen-Institut in Ulm, Germany, said they do not know why acupuncture works and plan more studies. "Acupuncture seems to be a useful tool for improving pregnancy rate after assisted reproductive techniques," they wrote. "The analysis shows that the pregnancy rate for the acupuncture group is considerably higher than for the control group (42.5% versus 26.3%)," they wrote.[1]

Working with a team at the Department of Chinese Medicine at Tongji Hospital in Wuhan, China, Paulus and colleagues tested 160 women undergoing *in vitro* fertilization. Half received the standard *in vitro* fertilization, while half were given acupuncture treatments before and after. "We chose acupuncture points that relax the uterus according to the principles of traditional Chinese medicine," they wrote. They said acupuncture can affect the autonomic nervous system—involved in the control of muscles and glands—and thus, theoretically, should make the lining of the uterus more receptive to receiving an embryo.

---

[1]Wolfgang E. Paulus, M.D., Mingmen Zhang, M.D., Erwin Strehler, M.D., Iman El-Danasouri, Ph.D., & Karl Sterzik, M.D., "Influence of acupuncture on the pregnancy rate in patients who undergo assisted reproduction therapy", *Fertility and Sterility*, Vol. 77, No. 4, Apr. 2002

According to the report, about 26% of women who did not receive acupuncture became pregnant, compared with nearly 43% of women who underwent the traditional Chinese therapy 25 minutes before and again 25 minutes after embryo transfer. There were no differences in age, number of transferred embryos, or the number of previous cycles between the two groups of patients. In this study, women received acupuncture along the spleen and stomach channels in an attempt to relax the uterus and improve the flow of energy to this region. They also received acupuncture needles in their ears to stabilize the endocrine system.

"The results demonstrate that acupuncture therapy improves pregnancy rate," concluded Dr. Paulus and colleagues. "However, more research is needed to determine whether the higher pregnancy rate among women receiving acupuncture was due to actual physiological or psychological effects," they added. "If these findings are confirmed, they may help us improve the odds for our IVF patients," Dr. Sandra Carson, president-elect of the American Society of Reproductive Medicine, said in a prepared statement after the publication of this study in *Fertility and Sterility*.

The points used in this study were:

25 minutes before embryo transfer: *Qi Hai* (CV 6), *Di Ji* (Sp 8), *Tai Chong* (Liv 3), *Bai Hui* (GV 20), *Gui Lai* (St 29)
25 minutes after embryo transfer: *Zu San Li* (St 36), *San Yin Jiao* (Sp 6), *Xue Hai* (Sp 10), *He Gu* (LI 4)

In addition the following auricular points were used: *Shen Men*, Uterus, Endocrine, and Brain.

Two needles were inserted in the right ear, the other two needles in the left ear. The four needles remained in the ears for 25 minutes. The side of the auricular acupuncture was changed after embryo transfer.

Appendix 2

Western Fertility Drugs

The following are some of the most commonly prescribed Western drugs in assisted reproductive technology clinics. Hopefully, these descriptions will help professional acupuncturists and practitioners of Chinese medicine better understand the intent and use of these medicines in their ART and IVF patients.

Pergonal

Pergonal® is a natural product containing both human FSH and LH, 75 or 150 international units of each per ampule, plus 10mg lactose. This material is extracted from the urine of postmenopausal women, carefully purified and then freeze-dried in sterile glass ampules where it is sealed until used. Pergonal was the first drug using the hormones FSH and LH. Since then, numerous drugs similar to Pergonal have come on the market. These drugs include Metrodin®, Humegon®, Fertinex®, Repronex®, Follistim®, and Gonal-F®. These drugs differ in how they are made and how they are administered. However, the comments concerning monitoring, risks, and other concerns are all the same regardless of which drug is used.

Pergonal is used to either induce or correct abnormalities of ovulation in women where other methods have been ineffective. It is also used to treat those women who are infertile, who have not conceived, and for whom *in vitro* fertilization would be the next step. This technique, called "controlled ovarian hyperstimulation" or COH, is often effective, particularly in couples with "minimal abnormality infertility," such as early endometriosis or similar problems.

To control ovulation in a normal menstrual cycle, the pituitary gland produces two hormones: FSH and LH. Pergonal is nothing more than a mixture of those two hormones. It is the natural hormones produced by a woman's pituitary gland. In a normal menstrual cycle, there are controls set up by the body to make sure that the number of eggs produced is limited (usually only one) and that the egg's maturity is optimum. The administration of Pergonal bypasses your body's natural control systems. Artificial control mechanisms must, therefore, be substituted and strict monitoring is necessary to reduce the likelihood of complications such as multiple pregnancies or hyperstimulation.

Because of the nature of the drug, it cannot be taken by mouth. The drug must, therefore, be given by injection. Pergonal injections are started on the 3rd day of the menstrual cycle. To insure maximum safety and efficiency of Pergonal, therapy must be constantly and carefully monitored. This is done using a combination of hormone levels and ultrasound examinations. In this way, the growth and development of the follicles within the ovary are monitored. Without such monitoring, Pergonal therapy can be dangerous.

There are two principal risks to Pergonal therapy. The first is "hyperstimulation syndrome." This occurs if the follicles are overstimulated *and* a shot of human chorionic gonadotropin (hCG) is then given to trigger ovulation. If the hCG shot is not given, hyperstimulation will not occur. Mild forms of hyperstimulation often occur even when the follicles are not overstimulated. Hyperstimulation may also occur if conception occurs in that cycle. Very thin women are more prone to hyperstimulation than women who are of normal weight or who are overweight. Women with irregular menstrual cycles are more prone to hyperstimulation than women with regular cycles. Women with Polycystic Ovarian Syndrome (PCOS) are often very sensitive and have to be monitored very carefully.

Serious hyperstimulation of the ovaries most often occurs if the estradiol (one of the subtypes of estrogen) level goes well over 2,000. If this happens, the whole cycle may be canceled. It also depends on the reason for the Pergonal therapy. Some groups of women are more likely to "hyperstimulate" than others. Symptoms of mild hyperstimulation include lower abdominal swelling and pain or discomfort in the region of the ovaries. Ultrasound examination will show enlargement of the ovaries with multiple cysts. Therapy for mild hyperstimulation involves nothing more than rest, avoidance of strenuous activity, and mild analgesics.

Repronex

Repronex® (menotropins for injection) is a purified preparation of gonadotropins extracted from the urine of postmenopausal women. Each vial of Repronex contains 75 or 150 IU of FSH activity and 75 or 150 IU of LH activity. Repronex is administered by subcutaneous or intramuscular injection. Repronex, in conjunction with hCG, is indicated for multiple follicular development (controlled ovarian stimulation) and ovulation induction in patients who have previously received pituitary suppression. Repronex is contraindicated in women who have:

1. A high FSH level indicating primary ovarian failure
2. Uncontrolled thyroid and adrenal dysfunction
3. An organic intracranial lesion such as a pituitary tumor
4. The presence of any cause of infertility other than anovulation unless they are candidates for *in vitro* fertilization
5. Abnormal bleeding of undetermined origin
6. Ovarian cysts or enlargement not due to polycystic ovary syndrome
7. Prior hypersensitivity to menotropins

Follistim

Follistim® (follitropin beta for injection) is the first recombinant follicle-stimulating hormone (FSH) to receive FDA approval in the United States for induction of ovulation in women experiencing anovulation (an absence of ovulation) and in women undergoing assisted reproductive technology (ART) procedures. Follistim was studied in the world's largest randomized *in vitro* fertilization study ever conducted. The study included 981 women undergoing IVF at 18 centers throughout Europe. The results demonstrated that Follistim is "safe and effective." Follistim acts like naturally produced FSH by stimulating the development of follicles within the ovary. It binds to the FSH receptors located on the surface of small granulosa cells surrounding the immature follicle and oocyte. However, Follistim does not induce ovulation. For ovulation to occur, therapy with Follistim is followed by a single administration of 5,000 to 10,000 IU of human chorionic gonadotropin (hCG). The dosage range for Follistim is 75-600 IU daily depending on the patient's response. Follistim may be administered either subcutaneously or intramuscularly. Although Follistim may cause certain adverse effects, the incidence of these events is relatively low and similar to that of other FSH-containing infertility products.

Gonal-F

Gonal-F® (follitropin alpha for injection) is a highly pure and consistent FSH produced by rDNA technology. Gonal-F acts directly on the ovaries to help stimulate the development of follicles. It is administered daily, and the length of treatment per cycle varies from patient to patient dependent on individual patient response to this drug. Gonal-F comes in an ampule that contains powder which needs to be mixed with sterile water. This medication is administered by easy subcutaneous injection, thus allowing for self-administration.

Clomid

Clomid® (clomiphene citrate, serophene) is a synthetic drug which stimulates the hypothalamus to release more GnRH. This, in turn, prompts the pituitary to release more LH and FSH and thus increases the stimulation of the ovary to begin to produce a mature egg. Clomid is a good first choice drug when a woman's ovaries are capable of functioning normally and when her hypothalamus and pituitary are also capable of producing their hormones. Structurally similar to estrogen, Clomid binds to the sites in the brain where estrogen normally attaches, called estrogen receptors. Once these receptor sites are filled up with clomiphene, they cannot bind with natural estrogen circulating in the blood and they are fooled into thinking that the amount of estrogen in the blood is too low. In response, the hypothalamus releases more GnRH, causing the pituitary to pump out more FSH which then causes a follicle to grow to produce more estrogen and start maturing an egg to prepare for ovulation. Typically, a woman taking Clomid produces double or triple the amount of estrogen in that cycle compared to pretreatment cycles.

If a woman is menstruating, even if irregularly, Clomid is usually effective, particularly if she develops follicles that are not reaching normal size. Usually, a mature follicle is about 20 millimeters in diameter or about the size of a small grape just before it ruptures and releases its egg. Clomid may help small, immature follicles grow to maturity. Clomid is also often effective for a woman with luteal phase defect (LPD). A woman with LPD may begin the ovulation process properly, but her ovarian function becomes disrupted, resulting in low production of the hormone progesterone in the luteal phase of the menstrual cycle. Following ovulation, the ovary produces progesterone, the hormone needed to prepare the uterine lining for implantation of the fertilized egg which has divided and entered the uterine cavity. A fall in progesterone levels in the blood during this critical time can interfere with early embryo implantation or, even if a fertilized egg has already implanted, cause a woman to menstruate too early and end a pregnancy within a few days after implantation.

If a woman responds to Clomid and develops a mature follicle (determined by adequate estrogen production and ultrasound examination) but has no LH surge by cycle day 15, then injection of hCG, which acts like LH, can be given to stimulate final egg maturation and follicle rupture, thus releasing the egg. The woman tends to ovulate about 36 hours after the LH surge or hCG injection. This can be confirmed by further ultrasound scans. If a woman does not ovulate after taking one Clomid tablet for five days, then her doctor will usually double the daily dose to two tablets (100mg) in her next cycle, and, if she still does not respond, then triple the daily dose to 150mg or add another fertility medication, such as Pergonal in the next cycle. Some doctors increase the dose up to 250mg a day, but this is not recommended by either of the drug's two manufacturers. Women tend to have side effects much more frequently at higher doses. If the dose of clomiphene is too high, the uterine lining may not respond completely to estrogen and progesterone stimulation and may not develop properly. As a result, a woman's fertilized egg may not be able to implant in her uterus.

Because Clomid binds to estrogen receptors, including the estrogen receptors in the cervix, it can interfere with the ability of the cervical mucus glands to be stimulated by estrogen to produce fertile mucus. Only "hostile" or dry cervical mucus may develop in the days preceding ovulation. If this occurs, adding a small amount of estrogen beginning on cycle day 10 and continuing until the LH surge may enhance cervical mucus production. Some women taking Clomid experience hot flashes and premenstrual-type symptoms, such as migraines and breast discomfort (particularly if they have fibrocystic disease of the breasts). Visual symptoms, such as spots, flashes, or blurry vision, are less common and indicate that treatment should stop.

Lupron

Lupron® (leuprolide) is a synthetic version of the naturally occurring gonadotropin-releasing hormone (GnRH) which is a hormone normally released from the hypothalamus. Lupron may be used for a number of different medical problems. These include treatment for prevention of premature LH surges with assisted reproductive technologies (ART); anemia caused by bleeding of uterine myomas; central precocious puberty (CPP); and pain due to endometriosis in women. In women, Lupron is given as a shot or nasal spray to lower one's estrogen level and, hopefully, suppress endometriosis. About 1-2 weeks after receiving her first dose, one enters a pseudo-menopausal state with low levels of estrogen, hot flashes, and other such menopausal side effects.

hCG

hCG stands for human chorionic gonadotropin, a polypeptide hormone produced by the human placenta. It is composed of an alpha and a beta subunit. The alpha subunit is essentially identical to the alpha subunits of the human pituitary gonadotropins, luteinizing hormone (LH) and follicle-stimulating hormone (FSH), as well as to the alpha sub-unit of human thyroid-stimulating hormone (TSH). The beta subunits of these hormones differ in amino acid sequence. Chorionic gonadotropin is obtained from the human pregnancy urine. It is used in fertility clinics to help stimulate the release of the egg. hCG is contraindicated in precocious puberty, prostatic carcinoma, or other androgen-dependent neoplasms, or in those with a prior allergic reaction to hCG. One well-known brand of hCG in the U.S. is Novarel® which is given by injection.

Prednisolone

Prednisolone is a cortisone-like drug which is sold in North America under a wide variety of names as well as being available as a generic in the U.S. and Canada. It is effective for relief of a wide variety of inflammatory and allergic disorders and is also effective in suppressing immunity. In the fertility clinic, it is used to suppress the immune system and, therefore, increase implantation as long as there is no antibody problem.

Estradiol

Estradiol is one of the estrogens or female sex hormones. Some of its common prescription names in the U.S. include Estrace®, Estraguard®, Estratab®, Gynetone®, PMS-Estradiol®, and Premarin®. In the fertility clinic, estradiol is used to help the endometrium become thicker for implantation and for the prevention of miscarriage, especially in women using an egg donor.

Progesterone

Progesterone is one of the steroid hormones. It is secreted by the corpus luteum and by the placenta and is responsible for preparing the body for pregnancy and, if pregnancy occurs, maintaining it until birth. Like all steroids, it is a small hydrophobic molecule. Thus it diffuses freely through the plasma membrane of all cells. However, in target cells, like those of the endometrium, it becomes tightly bound to a cytoplasmic protein, the progesterone receptor. Then the complex of receptor and its hormone moves into the nucleus where it binds to a progesterone response element. The progesterone response element is a specific sequence of DNA in the promoters of certain genes that is needed to turn those genes on (or off). Thus, the complex of progesterone with its receptor forms a transcription factor. In the fertility clinic, exogenous or supplemental progesterone is delivered by intramuscular (IM) injection or by vaginal suppository.

Progesterone is an important hormone in preventing miscarriage. Without adequate progesterone, the uterine lining will remain rigid, thereby, making pregnancy difficult to achieve. The lack of normal progesterone production by the ovaries in the second half of the menstrual cycle is called luteal phase defect. Women who have this defect either are unable to have their fertilized eggs implant in their uterine lining or, if the egg is implanted, it is so weak that miscarriage is a certain outcome.

To lessen the possibility of miscarriage, women who have a luteal phase defect use progesterone supplements after ovulation to help maximize the chance of carrying a pregnancy to full term. Progesterone supplements are also prescribed to women who are undergoing IVF and other methods of assisted reproductive technology. Progesterone supplements are given to women following an egg transfer in certain types of fertilization methods. Treatment for all women using progesterone supplements continues for at least 14 days following ovulation. If pregnancy occurs in a woman who is taking progesterone supplements, her doctor may decide to continue the treatment for another 8-10 weeks until placental autonomy occurs. Placental autonomy occurs when the placenta manufactures sufficient progesterone itself to support the pregnancy.

Antagon

Antagon Injection® (ganirelix acetate) is used to inhibit premature ovulation in women undergoing fertility procedures. It prevents the premature rise in levels of luteinizing hormone in women undergoing ovarian hyperstimulation as a part of specific infertility treatments such as IVF and ICSI (intracytoplasmic sperm injection). During stimulation of the growth of multiple follicles with gonadotropins, such as follicle-stimulating hormone (FSH), a rise in LH at too early a time may have unfavorable effects on the eggs and the possibility of getting pregnant. In general, there are two types of treatment regimens used to avoid an early rise in LH: GnRH-agonists and GnRH-antagonists. Antagon is a GnRH-antagonist that has the ability to rapidly inhibit LH release instantaneously. It achieves quickly what GnRH-agonists can take 2-3 weeks to do and is, therefore, only required during the final days of stimulation. However, women who have experienced a hypersensitivity reaction to gonadotropin-releasing hormone (GnRH) or any other GnRH-type drug and/or women who suspect or know they are pregnant should not use Antagon. The most frequent side effects of Antagon are abdominal pain, fetal death, and headache.

Baby Aspirin

A study, which was conducted by following the history of over 1,000 women, has indicated that women who suffer unexplained late recurrent miscarriages may benefit from a daily, low dose aspirin (acetylsalicylic acid, 75mg tablet). The birth rate in this group was 65% compared with 49% in the women who did not take aspirin. Antiphospholipid antibody syndrome is a clinical sequence of events that affects clotting and may cause recurrent pregnancy loss and low platelets. Two autoantibodies are involved in this condition: the lupus anticoagulant (LAC) and anticardiolipin antibody (ACA). Some clinicians are convinced that antiphospholipid antibodies are associated with infertility as well and, in some cases, women are treated with heparin to improve the rate of pregnancy. In the treatment of recurrent miscarriage, where ACA and/or LAC is suspected, it has been found that heparin plus low dose aspirin (80-100mg per day) is beneficial. Moderate severity of disease is more responsive to aspirin therapy than are the more severe cases. Baby aspirin is used because of its smaller dosage.

Appendix 3

Chinese Medicinals

The following are thumbnail sketches of the Chinese medicinals described in the text. They are given for those who are less familiar with these medicinals. Included are standard dosage ranges when used in decoction. The exact dose of any medicinal in any formula in this text is dependent on three factors: 1) the role the medicinal plays in the formula, 2) the patient's particular needs, and 3) the characteristic range for that medicinal. The following medicinals are arranged according to their standard categorization and from commonly used to less commonly used in the protocols contained herein.

Yin-supplementing medicinals

Han Lian Cao (Herba Ecliptae Prostratae)

Nature & flavor: Sweet, sour, cool
Channels entered: Liver, kidney
Functions:
1. Nourishes and supplements the liver and kidneys
2. Cools the blood and stops bleeding
Dosage: 9-15g

Nu Zhen Zi (Fructus Ligustri Lucidi)

Nature & flavor: Bitter, sweet, neutral
Channels entered: Liver, kidney
Functions:
1. Nourishes and supplements the liver and kidneys
2. Supplements the kidneys and clears vacuity heat

3. Nourishes the liver and brightens the eyes
Dosage: 4.5-15g

Sang Ji Sheng (Ramulus Sangjisheng)

Nature & flavor: Bitter, neutral
Channels entered: Kidney, liver
Functions:
1. Supplements the liver and kidneys, strengthens the sinews and bones
2. Nourishes the blood and quiets the fetus
3. Nourishes the blood and moistens the skin
Dosage: 12-40g

Mai Men Dong (Tuber Ophiopogonis Japonici)

Nature & flavor: Sweet, slightly bitter, slightly cold
Channels entered: Heart, lung, spleen
Functions:
1. Moistens the lungs and stops cough
2. Boosts the stomach and engenders fluids
3. Clears the heart and eliminates vexation
4. Moistens the intestines
Dosage: 9-15g

Tian Men Dong (Tuber Asparagi Cochinensis)

Nature & flavor: Sweet, bitter, very cold
Channels entered: Kidney, lung
Functions:
1. Nourishes yin and clears the lungs
2. Moistens the lungs, nourishes the kidneys, and generates fluids
Dosage: 6-15g

Sha Shen (Radix Glehniae Littoralis)

Nature & flavor: Bland, cool
Channels entered: Lung, stomach
Functions:
1. Moistens the lungs and stops coughing

2. Nourishes the stomach and generates fluids
3. Moistens the exterior
Dosage: 9-15g

Yang-supplementing medicinals

Xu Duan (Radix Dipsaci Asperi)

Nature & flavor: Bitter, acrid, slightly warm
Channels entered: Liver, kidney
Functions:
1. Supplements the liver and kidneys, strengthens the sinews and bones
2. Stops uterine bleeding and quiets the fetus
3. Quickens the blood, alleviates pain, and generates flesh
Dosage: 6-24g

Du Zhong (Cortex Eucommiae Ulmoidis)

Nature & flavor: Sweet, slightly acrid, warm
Channels entered: Liver, kidney
Functions:
1. Supplements the liver and kidneys, strengthens the sinews and bones
2. Promotes the smooth and free flow of qi and blood
3. Quiets the fetus
Dosage: 6-15g

Tu Si Zi (Semen Cuscutae Chinensis)

Nature & flavor: Acrid, sweet, warm
Channels entered: Liver, kidney
Functions:
1. Supplements the kidneys and fosters the essence
2. Supplements the liver and kidneys and improves vision
3. Fortifies the spleen, supplements the kidneys, and stops diarrhea
4. Quiets the fetus
Dosage: 9-15g

Ba Ji Tian (Radix Morindae Officinalis)

Nature & flavor: Acrid, sweet, warm
Channels entered: Liver, kidney
Functions:
1. Supplements the kidneys and invigorates yang
2. Strengthens the sinews and bones
3. Courses wind and dispels dampness and cold
Dosage: 9-15g

Yin Yang Huo (Herba Epimedii)

Nature & flavor: Acrid, sweet, warm
Channels entered: Liver, kidney
Functions:
1. Supplements the kidneys and invigorates yang
2. Expels wind, cold, and dampness and alleviates pain
3. Supplements yin and yang and downbears liver yang
Dosage: 6-15g

Rou Cong Rong (Herba Cistanchis Deserticolae)

Nature & flavor: Sweet, salty, warm
Channels entered: Large intestine, kidney
Functions:
1. Supplements the kidneys and invigorates yang
2. Warms the uterus
3. Moistens the intestines and frees the flow of the stools
Dosage: 9-21g

Bu Gu Zhi (Fructus Psoraleae Corylifoliae)

Nature & flavor: Acrid, bitter, very warm
Channels entered: Kidney, spleen
Functions:
1. Supplements the kidneys and invigorates yang
2. Secures the essence
3. Fortifies the spleen and warms yang
4. Promotes the kidneys' absorption of the qi
Dosage: 3-9g

Suo Yang (Herba Cynomorii Songarici)

Nature & flavor: Sweet, warm
Channels entered: Large intestine, kidney, liver
Functions:
1. Supplements the kidneys and invigorates yang
2. Nourishes the blood and boosts the essence
3. Moistens the intestines and frees the flow of the stools
Dosage: 4.5-15g

Yi Zhi Ren (Fructus Alpiniae Oxyphyllae)

Nature & flavor: Acrid, warm
Channels entered: Kidney, spleen
Functions:
1. Warms the kidneys and secures the essence
2. Warms the spleen and stops diarrhea
Dosage: 3-9g

Zi He Che (Placenta Hominis)

Nature & flavor: Sweet, salty, warm
Channels entered: Liver, lung, kidney
Functions:
1. Supplements the liver and kidneys and boosts the essence
2. Supplements the qi and nourishes the blood
3. Supplements the lung qi and boosts kidney essence
Dosage: 1.5-4.5g

Yang Qi Shi (Actinolitum)

Nature & flavor: Salty, slightly warm
Channels entered: Kidney
Functions:
1. Warms the kidneys and invigorates yang
2. Warms the uterus
Dosage: 3-4.5g

Lu Jiao (Cornu Cervi)

Nature & flavor: Sweet, salty, warm
Channels entered: Liver, kidney
Functions:
1. Supplements the kidneys and invigorates yang
2. Supplements the governing vessel and boosts the essence
3. Regulates and rectifies the thoroughfare and controlling vessels
4. Supplements and nourishes the qi and blood
Dosage: 1-3g

Securing & astringing medicinals

Shan Zhu Yu (Fructus Corni Officinalis)

Nature & flavor: Sour, slightly warm
Channels entered: Liver, kidney
Functions:
1. Secures the kidneys and astringes the essence
2. Stops sweating and stems desertion
3. Supplements and boosts the liver and kidneys
4. Secures the menses and stops bleeding
Dosage: 4.5-9g

Wu Wei Zi (Fructus Schisandrae Chinensis)

Nature & flavor: Sour, warm
Channels entered: Large intestine, liver, lung, spleen
Functions:
1. Secures the lungs and stops coughing
2. Supplements the kidneys and secures the essence
3. Generates fluids and stops sweating
4. Quiets the heart and calms the spirit
Dosage: 1.5-9g

Jin Ying Zi (Fructus Rosae Laevigatae)

Nature & flavor: Sour, astringent, neutral
Channels entered: Bladder, kidney, large intestine

Functions:
1. Hardens the kidneys and secures the essence
2. Secures the intestines and stops diarrhea
Dosage: 4.5-9g

Qian Shi (Semen Euryalis Ferocis)

Nature & flavor: Sweet, astringent, neutral
Channels entered: Kidney, spleen
Functions:
1. Fortifies the spleen and stops diarrhea
2. Hardens the kidneys and secures the essence
3. Eliminates dampness and stops abnormal vaginal discharge
Dosage: 9-15g

Hai Piao Xiao (Os Sepiae Seu Sepiellae)

Nature & flavor: Salty, astringent, slightly warm
Channels entered: Kidney, liver, stomach
Functions:
1. Stops bleeding and abnormal vaginal discharge
2. Secures the essence
3. Absorbs acidity and alleviates pain
4. Stops diarrhea
Dosage: 4.5-12g

Qi-supplementing medicinals

Ren Shen (Radix Panacis Ginseng)

Nature & flavor: Sweet, slightly bitter, slightly warm
Channels entered: Lung, spleen
Functions:
1. Strongly supplements the source qi
2. Supplements the lungs and boosts the qi
3. Fortifies the spleen and supplements the stomach
4. Generates fluids and alleviates thirst
5. Boosts the heart qi and quiets the spirit
Dosage: 1-9g

Dang Shen (Radix Codonopsitis Pilosulae)

Nature & flavor: Sweet, neutral
Channels entered: Lung, spleen
Functions:
1. Supplements the middle burner and boosts the qi
2. Supplements the lungs
3. Supplements the qi and nourishes fluids
Dosage: 9-30g

Bai Zhu (Rhizoma Atractylodis Macrocephalae)

Nature & flavor: Bitter, sweet, warm
Channels entered: Spleen, stomach
Functions:
1. Fortifies the spleen and boosts the qi
2. Fortifies the spleen and dries dampness
3. Secures the exterior and stops sweating
4. Fortifies the spleen and quiets the fetus
Dosage: 4.5-15g

Gan Cao (Radix Glycyrrhizae Uralanesis)

Nature & flavor: Sweet, neutral
Channels entered: All 12
Functions:
1. Fortifies the spleen and boosts the qi
2. Moistens the lungs and stops coughing
3. Clears heat and resolves toxins
4. Relaxes spasms and alleviates pain
5. Moderates and harmonizes the characteristics of other medicinals
Dosage: 4.5-9g

Huang Qi (Radix Astragali Membranacei)

Nature & flavor: Sweet, slightly warm
Channels entered: Lung, spleen
Functions:
1. Fortifies the spleen and boosts the qi

2. Upbears yang of the spleen and stomach
3. Supplements the defensive qi and secures the exterior
4. Supplements the qi and blood
5. Seeps water and disperses swelling
6. Promotes the discharge of pus and generates flesh
Dosage: 9-60g

Shan Yao (Radix Dioscoreae Oppositae)

Nature & flavor: Sweet, neutral
Channels entered: Kidney, lung, spleen
Functions:
1. Supplements and boosts the spleen and stomach
2. Supplements the lung qi and boosts lung yin
3. Supplements the kidneys, secures and astringes
Dosage: 9-30g

Da Zao (Fructus Ziziphi Jujubae)

Nature & flavor: Sweet, neutral
Channels entered: Spleen, stomach
Functions:
1. Fortifies the spleen and boosts the qi
2. Nourishes the blood and quiets the spirit
3. Moderates and harmonizes the harsh properties of other medicinals
Dosage: 3-12 pieces

Huang Jing (Rhizoma Polygonati)

Nature & flavor: Sweet, neutral
Channels entered: Kidney, lung, spleen
Functions:
1. Supplements spleen qi and enriches spleen yin
2. Moistens the lungs
3. Supplements the kidneys and fosters the essence
4. Treats wasting thirst
Dosage: 9-21g

Blood-supplementing medicinals

Bai Shao (Radix Albus Paeoniae Lactiflorae)

Nature & flavor: Bitter, sour, cool
Channels entered: Liver, spleen
Functions:
1. Nourishes the blood and regulates menstruation
2. Emolliates the liver and alleviates pain
3. Preserves liver yin and subdues liver yang
Dosage: 4.5-30g

Gou Qi Zi (Fructus Lycii Chinensis)

Nature & flavor: Sweet, neutral
Channels entered: Liver, lung, kidney
Functions:
1. Nourishes and supplements the liver and kidneys
2. Fosters the essence and brightens the eyes
3. Enriches yin and moistens the lungs
Dosage: 6-18g

Dang Gui (Radix Angelicae Sinensis)

Nature & flavor: Sweet, acrid, warm
Channels entered: Heart, liver, spleen
Functions:
1. Supplements the blood and regulates menstruation
2. Moistens the intestines and frees the flow of the stools
3. Disperses swelling, expels pus, generates flesh, and alleviates pain
Dosage: 4.5-15g

Shu Di Huang (cooked Radix Rehmanniae Glutinosae)

Nature & flavor: Sweet, slightly warm
Channels entered: Heart, kidney, liver
Functions:
1. Supplements the blood
2. Nourishes yin

3. Nourishes the blood and supplements the essence
Dosage: 9-30g

He Shou Wu (Radix Polygoni Multiflori)

Nature & flavor: Bitter, sweet, astringent, slightly warm
Channels entered: Liver, kidney
Functions:
1. Supplements the liver and kidneys, nourishes the blood and boosts the essence
2. Secures the essence and stops leakage
3. Clears heat and resolves toxins
4. Moistens the intestines and frees the flow of the stools
Dosage: 9-30g

Sang Shen Zi (Fructus Mori Albi)

Nature & flavor: Sweet, cold
Channels entered: Heart, liver, kidney
Functions: Supplements the blood and enriches yin
Dosage: 6-15g

Long Yan Rou (Arillus Euphoriae Longanae)

Nature & flavor: Sweet, warm
Channels entered: Heart, spleen
Functions: Supplements and boosts the heart and spleen
Dosage: 6-15g

E Jiao (Gelatinum Corii Asini)

Nature & flavor: Sweet, neutral
Channels entered: Kidney, liver, lung
Functions:
1. Nourishes the blood and enriches yin
2. Stops bleeding
Dosage: 3-15g

Acrid, warm exterior-resolving medicinals

Gui Zhi (Ramulus Cinnamomi Cassiae)

Nature & flavor: Acrid, sweet, warm
Channels entered: Heart, lung, bladder
Functions:
1. Harmonizes the constructive and defensive aspects
2. Warms the channels and dispels cold
3. Frees the flow of yang and transforms the qi
4. Warms and loosens the chest qi
5. Warms and quickens the blood vessels (or blood and vessels)
Dosage: 3-9g

Fang Feng (Radix Ledebouriellae Divaricatae)

Nature & flavor: Sweet, slightly warm
Channels entered: Bladder, liver, spleen
Functions:
1. Resolves the exterior and dispels wind
2. Expels wind and dampness and alleviates pain
3. Harmonizes the liver and spleen
Dosage: 3-9g

Jing Jie Sui (Herba Seu Flos Schizonepetae Tenuifoliae)

Nature & flavor: Acrid, aromatic, slightly warm
Channels entered: Lung, liver
Functions:
1. Resolves the exterior and expels wind
2. Out-thrusts rashes and alleviates itching
3. Stops bleeding
Dosage: 3-9g

Sheng Jiang (uncooked Rhizoma Zingiberis Officinalis)

Nature & flavor: Acrid, warm
Channels entered: Lung, spleen, stomach
Functions:
1. Resolves the exterior and dispels cold

2. Warms the middle and alleviates vomiting
3. Dispels cold and stops coughing
4. Reduces the toxicity of other herbs
5. Harmonizes the constructive and defensive aspects
Dosage: 1-3 slices

Bai Zhi (Radix Angelicae Dahuricae)

Nature & flavor: Acrid, warm
Channels entered: Lung, stomach
Functions:
1. Dispels wind and alleviates pain
2. Disperses swelling and expels pus
3. Dispels dampness and stops discharge
4. Opens the orifices and frees the flow of the nose
Dosage: 3-9g

Acrid, cool exterior-resolving medicinals

Chai Hu (Radix Bupleuri)

Nature & flavor: Bitter, acrid, cool
Channels entered: Gallbladder, liver, pericardium, triple burner
Functions:
1. Resolves the *shao yang* and abates fever
2. Courses the liver and rectifies the qi
3. Upbears yang of the spleen and stomach
Dosage: 3-9g

Sang Ye (Folium Mori Albi)

Nature & flavor: Sweet, bitter, cold
Channels entered: Liver, lung
Functions:
1. Dispels wind and clears heat from the lungs
2. Clears the liver and brightens the eyes
3. Cools the blood and stops bleeding
Dosage: 4.5-15g

Ju Hua (Flos Chrysanthemi Morifolii)

Nature & flavor: Sweet, bitter, slightly cold
Channels entered: Liver, lung
Functions:
1. Dispels wind and clears heat
2. Clears the liver and brightens the eyes
3. Settles the liver and extinguishes wind
Dosage: 4.5-15g

Bo He (Herba Menthae Haplocalysis)

Nature & flavor: Acrid, aromatic, cool
Channels entered: Lung, liver
Functions:
1. Dispels wind and clears heat
2. Clears the head and eyes and disinhibits the throat
3. Out-thrusts rashes
4. Courses the liver and rectifies the qi
Dosage: 3-6g

Sheng Ma (Rhizoma Cimicifugae)

Nature & flavor: Sweet, acrid, cool
Channels entered: Large intestine, lung, spleen, stomach
Functions:
1. Resolves the exterior and out-thrusts rashes
2. Clears heat and resolves toxins
3. Upbears yang and lifts the fallen
Dosage: 1.5-9g

Qi-rectifying medicinals

Chen Pi (Pericarpium Citri Reticulatae)

Nature & flavor: Acrid, bitter, warm, aromatic
Channels entered: Lung, spleen, stomach
Functions:
1. Rectifies the qi, harmonizes the middle, and relaxes the diaphragm

2. Dries dampness and transforms phlegm
3. Helps prevent stagnation
Dosage: 3-9g

Xiang Fu (Rhizoma Cyperi Rotundi)

Nature & flavor: Acrid, slightly bitter, slightly sweet, neutral
Channels entered: Liver, triple burner
Functions:
1. Courses the liver and rectifies the qi
2. Regulates menstruation and alleviates pain
Dosage: 6-12g

Zhi Ke (Fructus Citri Aurantii)

Nature & flavor: Bitter, cool
Channels entered: Spleen, stomach
Functions: Moves the qi and disperses distention
Dosage: 3-15g

Wu Yao (Radix Linderae Strychnifoliae)

Nature & flavor: Acrid, warm
Channels entered: Bladder, kidney, lung, spleen
Functions:
1. Moves the qi and alleviates pain
2. Supplements the kidneys and warms yang
Dosage: 3-9g

Qing Pi (Pericarpium Citri Reticulatae Viride)

Nature & flavor: Bitter, acrid, warm
Channels entered: Gallbladder, liver, stomach
Functions:
1. Courses the liver and rectifies the qi
2. Disperses accumulations and stagnation
3. Dries dampness and transforms phlegm
Dosage: 3-9g

Mu Xiang (Radix Auklandiae Lappae)

Nature & flavor: Acrid, bitter, warm
Channels entered: Gallbladder, large intestine
Functions:
1. Moves the qi and alleviates pain
2. Harmonizes the stomach and intestines
3. Fortifies the spleen and prevents stagnation
Dosage: 1.5-9g

Li Zhi He (Semen Litchi Chinensis)

Nature & flavor: Sweet, astringent, warm
Channels entered: Liver, stomach
Functions:
1. Rectifies the qi and alleviates pain
2. Scatters cold and disperses stagnation
Dosage: 6-15g

Aromatic, dampness-transforming medicinals

Sha Ren (Fructus Amomi)

Nature & flavor: Acrid, warm, aromatic
Channels entered: Spleen, stomach
Functions:
1. Transforms dampness and stops vomiting
2. Moves the qi and fortifies the stomach
3. Quiets the fetus
Dosage: 1.5-6g

Cang Zhu (Rhizoma Atractylodis)

Nature & flavor: Acrid, bitter, warm, aromatic
Channels entered: Spleen, stomach
Functions:
1. Strongly dries dampness and fortifies the spleen
2. Dispels wind dampness
3. Eliminates dampness from the lower burner
4. Resolves the exterior and promotes sweating
Dosage: 4.5-9g

Hou Po (Cortex Magnoliae Officinalis)

Nature & flavor: Bitter, acrid, warm, aromatic
Channels entered: Large intestine, lung, spleen, stomach
Functions:
1. Moves the qi, transforms dampness, and disperses stagnation
2. Warms and transforms phlegm and downbears counterflow
Dosage: 3-9g

Dampness-seeping medicinals

Fu Ling (Sclerotuim Poriae Cocos)

Nature & flavor: Sweet, bland, neutral
Channels entered: Heart, spleen, lung, kidney
Functions:
1. Seeps dampness and frees the flow of urination
2. Fortifies the spleen and harmonizes the middle
3. Fortifies the spleen and transforms phlegm
4. Quiets the heart and calms the spirit
Dosage: 9-15g

Yi Yi Ren (Semen Coicis Lachryma-jobi)

Nature & flavor: Sweet, bland, slightly cold
Channels entered: Spleen, lung, kidney
Functions:
1. Seeps dampness and disinhibits urination
2. Fortifies the spleen and stops diarrhea
3. Clears heat and expels pus
4. Dispels wind, eliminates dampness, and alleviates pain
5. Clears heat and eliminates dampness
Dosage: 9-30g

Ze Xie (Rhizoma Alismatis Orientalitis)

Nature & flavor: Sweet, bland, cold
Channels entered: Kidney, bladder
Functions:
1. Seeps dampness and disinhibits urination

2. Drains kidney fire
Dosage: 4.5-9g

Che Qian Zi (Semen Plantaginis)

Nature & flavor: Sweet, cold
Channels entered: Bladder, kidney, liver, lung
Functions:
1. Disinhibits urination and clears heat
2. Disinhibits urination to solidify the stools
3. Brightens the eyes
4. Expels phlegm and stops cough
Dosage: 4.5-9g

Qu Mai (Herba Dianthi)

Nature & flavor: Bitter, cold
Channels entered: Bladder, heart, small intestine
Functions:
1. Clears and eliminates damp heat, disinhibits urination and frees the flow of strangury
2. Quickens the blood and dispels stasis
3. Frees the flow of the stools
Dosage: 3-9g

Zhu Ling (Sclerotium Polypori Umbellati)

Nature & flavor: Sweet, bland, slightly cool
Channels entered: Spleen, kidney, bladder
Functions: Seeps dampness and disinhibits urination
Dosage: 6-15g

Mu Tong (Caulis Akebiae)

Nature & flavor: Bitter, cool
Channels entered: Bladder, heart, small intestine
Functions:
1. Disinhibits urination and drains the heart

2. Frees the flow of the breasts (and/or milk)
3. Quickens the blood and frees the flow of the vessels
Dosage: 3-9g

Cold-warming, phlegm-transforming medicinals

Ban Xia (Rhizoma Pinelliae Ternatae)

Nature & flavor: Acrid, warm, toxic
Channels entered: Lung, spleen, stomach
Functions:
1. Dries dampness, transforms phlegm, and downbears counterflow
2. Harmonizes the stomach and stops vomiting
3. Scatters nodules and disperses distention
Dosage: 4.5-9g

Jie Geng (Radix Platycodi Grandiflori)

Nature & flavor: Bitter, acrid, neutral
Channels entered: Lung
Functions:
1. Diffuses and depurates the lung qi and expels phlegm
2. Promotes the discharge of pus
3. Disinhibits the throat
4. Guides the effect of other herbs to the upper regions of the body
Dosage: 3-9g

Heat-clearing, phlegm-transforming medicinals

Chuan Bei Mu (Bulbus Fritillariae Cirrhosae)

Nature & flavor: Bitter, sweet, slightly cold
Channels entered: Heart, lung
Functions:
1. Clears heat and transforms phlegm
2. Clears heat and scatters nodulation
Dosage: 3-12g

Hai Zao (Herba Sargassii)

Nature & flavor: Bitter, salty, cold
Channels entered: Kidney, liver, lung, stomach
Functions:
1. Clears heat and transforms phlegm
2. Softens the hard and scatters nodulation
3. Disinhibits urination and disperses swelling
Dosage: 4.5-15g

Kun Bu (Thallus Algae)

Nature & flavor: Salty, cold
Channels entered: Kidney, liver, stomach
Functions:
1. Transforms phlegm and scatters nodulation
2. Disinhibits urination and disperses swelling
Dosage: 4.5-15g

Tian Hua Fen (Radix Trichosanthis Kirlowii)

Nature & flavor: Bitter, slightly sweet, cold
Channels entered: Lung, stomach
Functions:
1. Clears the lungs and drains heat
2. Transforms phlegm and moistens dryness
3. Drains heat and generates fluids
4. Resolves toxins and expels pus
Dosage: 9-15g

Dan Nan Xing (bile-processed Rhizoma Arisaematis)

Nature & flavor: Bitter, cool
Channels entered: Liver, lung, spleen
Functions:
1. Clears heat and transforms phlegm
2. Extinguishes wind and resolves tetany
Dosage: 3-6g

Heat-clearing, fire-draining medicinals

Lu Gen (Rhizoma Phragmitis Communis)

Nature & flavor: Sweet, cold
Channels entered: Lung, stomach
Functions:
1. Clears heat and generates fluids
2. Clears heat from the lungs
3. Clears heat from the stomach
4. Clears heat and disinhibits urination
5. Out-thrusts rashes
Dosage: 6-30g

Zhi Zi (Fructus Gardeniae Jasminoidis)

Nature & flavor: Bitter, cold
Channels entered: Heart, liver, lung, stomach, triple burner
Functions:
1. Clears heat and eliminates vexation
2. Clears and eliminates dampness and heat
3. Cools the blood and stops bleeding
4. Quickens the blood and disperses swelling
Dosage: 3-12g

Heat-clearing, dampness-drying medicinals

Huang Qin (Radix Scutellariae Baicalensis)

Nature & flavor: Bitter, cold
Channels entered: Gallbladder, large intestine, lung, stomach
Functions:
1. Clears heat and drains fire, especially from the upper burner
2. Clears heat and dries dampness
3. Clears heat and stops bleeding
4. Clears heat and quiets the fetus
5. Clears the liver and drains yang
Dosage: 6-15g

Huang Bai (Cortex Phellodendri)

Nature & flavor: Bitter, cold
Channels entered: Kidney, bladder
Functions:
1. Clears and eliminates dampness and heat, particularly from the lower burner
2. Drains kidney fire
3. Drains fire and resolves toxins
Dosage: 3-12g

Heat-clearing, toxin-resolving medicinals

Jin Yin Hua (Flos Lonicerae Japonicae)

Nature & flavor: Sweet, cold
Channels entered: Large intestine, lung, stomach
Functions:
1. Clears heat and resolves toxins
2. Resolves the exterior and clears heat
3. Clears and eliminates dampness and heat from the lower burner
Dosage: 6-15g

Lian Qiao (Fructus Forsythiae Suspensae)

Nature & flavor: Bitter, slightly acrid, cool
Channels entered: Heart, liver, gallbladder
Functions:
1. Clears heat, resolves toxins, and scatters nodulation
2. Resolves the exterior and clears heat
Dosage: 3-15g

Zi Hua Di Ding (Herba Violae Yedoensitis Cum Radice)

Nature & flavor: Acrid, bitter, cold
Channels entered: Heart, liver
Functions: Clears heat and resolves toxins
Dosage: 9-15g

Yu Xing Cao (Herba Houttuyniae Cordatae Cum Radice)

Nature & flavor: Acrid, cool
Channels entered: Large intestine, lung
Functions:
1. Clears heat and resolves toxins
2. Resolves toxins and expels pus
3. Clears and eliminates dampness and heat and disinhibits urination
Dosage: 15-60g

Bai Hua She She Cao (Herba Oldenlandiae Diffusae)

Nature & flavor: Bitter, sweet, cold
Channels entered: Liver, stomach, large intestine
Functions:
1. Clears heat and resolves toxins
2. Clears heat and eliminates dampness via disinhibiting urination
Dosage: 15-60g

Heat-clearing, blood-cooling medicinals

Mu Dan Pi (Cortex Radicis Moutan)

Nature & flavor: Acrid, bitter, cool
Channels entered: Heart, liver, kidney
Functions:
1. Clears heat and cools the blood
2. Clears vacuity heat
3. Quickens the blood and dispels stasis
4. Clears the liver and drains yang
5. Drains pus and disperses swelling
Dosage: 6-12g

Sheng Di Huang (uncooked Radix Rehmanniae Glutinosae)

Nature & flavor: Sweet, bitter, cold
Channels entered: Heart, kidney, liver
Functions:
1. Clears heat and cools the blood

2. Nourishes yin and generates fluids
3. Clears upward blazing of heart fire
Dosage: 9-30g

Xuan Shen (Radix Scrophulariae Ningpoensis)

Nature & flavor: Salty, sweet, bitter, cold
Channels entered: Kidney, lung, stomach
Functions:
1. Clears heat and cools the blood
2. Nourishes yin
3. Drains fire and resolves toxins
4. Softens the hard and scatters nodulation
Dosage: 9-30g

Di Gu Pi (Cortex Radicis Lycii Chinensis)

Nature & flavor: Sweet, cold
Channels entered: Lung, liver, kidney
Functions:
1. Clears vacuity heat
2. Clears heat and stops coughing
3. Clears heat and cools the blood
Dosage: 6-15g

Heat-clearing, summerheat-resolving medicinals

Qing Hao (Herba Artemisiae Annuae)

Nature & flavor: Bitter, cold
Channels entered: Kidney, liver, gallbladder
Functions:
1. Clears summerheat
2. Clears vacuity heat
3. Cools the blood and stops bleeding
4. Treats malaria-like disorders
Dosage: 3-9g

Interior-warming, cold-dispelling medicinals

Gan Jiang (dry Rhizoma Zingiberis Officinalis)

Nature & flavor: Acrid, hot
Channels entered: Heart, lung, spleen, stomach
Functions:
1. Warms the middle and scatters cold
2. Rescues yang and warms the interior
3. Warms the lungs and transforms phlegm
4. Warms the channels and stops bleeding
Dosage: 3-12g

Rou Gui (Cortex Cinnamomi Cassiae)

Nature & flavor: Acrid, sweet, hot
Channels entered: Heart, kidney, liver, spleen
Functions:
1. Warms the kidneys and invigorates yang
2. Guides fire back to its lower source
3. Dispels cold and warms the channels, frees the flow of the channels and vessels and alleviates pain
4. Promotes the engenderment and transformation of qi and blood
Dosage: 1.5-4.5g

Xiao Hui Xiang (Fructus Foeniculi Vulgaris)

Nature & flavor: Acrid, warm
Channels entered: Liver, kidney, spleen, stomach
Functions:
1. Courses the liver and warms the kidneys, dispels cold and alleviates pain
2. Rectifies the qi and harmonizes the stomach
Dosage: 3-9g

Chuan Jiao (Pericarpium Zanthoxyli Bungeani)

Nature & flavor: Acrid, hot, slightly toxic
Channels entered: Kidney, spleen, stomach
Functions:
1. Warms the middle, dispels cold, and alleviates pain
2. Kills worms and alleviates pain
Dosage: 1.5-6g

Wind dampness treating medicinal

Du Huo (Radix Angelicae Pubescentis)

Nature & flavor: Bitter, acrid, warm
Channels entered: Kidney, bladder
Functions:
1. Dispels wind, eliminates dampness, and alleviates pain
2. Resolves the exterior and dispels wind, cold, and dampness
3. Also used for *shao yin* headache and toothache
Dosage: 3-9g

Blood-quickening medicinals

Dan Shen (Radix Salviae Miltiorrhizae)

Nature & flavor: Bitter, slightly cold
Channels entered: Heart, pericardium, liver
Functions:
1. Quickens the blood and transforms stasis
2. Clears heat and eliminates vexation
Dosage: 4.5-15g

Hong Hua (Flos Carthami Tinctorii)

Nature & flavor: Acrid, warm
Channels entered: Heart, liver
Functions:
1. Quickens the blood and frees the flow of menstruation
2. Dispels stasis and alleviates pain
Dosage: 3-9g

Chuan Xiong (Radix Ligustici Wallichii)

Nature & flavor: Acrid, warm
Channels entered: Liver, gallbladder, pericardium
Functions:
1. Moves the qi within the blood, thereby quickening the blood and dispelling stasis
2. Expels wind and alleviates pain
3. Treats headache
Dosage: 3-9g

Niu Xi (Radix Achyranthis Bidentatae)

Nature & flavor: Bitter, sour, neutral
Channels entered: Liver, kidney
Functions:
1. Quickens the blood and dispels stasis
2. Strengthens the sinews and bones and disinhibits the joints
3. Clears and eliminates dampness and heat from the lower burner
4. Guides the blood and moves it downward
Dosage: 6-15g

Yi Mu Cao (Herba Leonuri Heterophylli)

Nature & flavor: Acrid, bitter, slightly cold
Channels entered: Heart, liver, bladder
Functions:
1. Quickens the blood and regulates menstruation
2. Quickens the blood and disperses concretions
3. Disinhibits urination and disperses swelling
Dosage: 9-30g

Tao Ren (Semen Pruni Persicae)

Nature & flavor: Bitter, sweet, neutral
Channels entered: Heart, large intestine, liver, lung
Functions:
1. Quickens the blood and dispels stasis
2. Moistens the intestines and frees the flow of the stools
Dosage: 6-9g

Ji Xue Teng (Radix Et Caulis Jixueteng)

Nature & flavor: Bitter, sweet, warm
Channels entered: Heart, liver, spleen
Functions:
1. Quickens and nourishes the blood
2. Frees the flow of the channels and relaxes the sinews
3. Supplements the blood and quickens the channels
Dosage: 9-15g

E Zhu (Rhizoma Curcumae Ezhu)

Nature & flavor: Bitter, acrid, warm
Channels entered: Liver, spleen
Functions:
1. Breaks the blood, moves the qi, and alleviates pain
2. Disperses accumulations and alleviates pain
Dosage: 3-9g

Chi Shao (Radix Rubrus Paeoniae Lactiflorae)

Nature & flavor: Sour, bitter, slightly cold
Channels entered: Liver, spleen
Functions:
1. Quickens the blood and dispels stasis
2. Clears heat and cools the blood
3. Clears the liver and drains fire
Dosage: 4.5-9g

San Leng (Rhizoma Sparganii Stoloniferi)

Nature & flavor: Bitter, acrid, neutral
Channels entered: Liver, spleen
Functions:
1. Forcefully breaks the blood, moves the qi, and alleviates pain
2. Disperses accumulations
Dosage: 3-9g

Ru Xiang (Resina Olibani)

Nature & flavor: Acrid, bitter, warm
Channels entered: Heart, liver, spleen
Functions:
1. Quickens the blood and moves the qi
2. Relaxes the sinews, quickens the channels, and alleviates pain
3. Disperses swelling and generates flesh
Dosage: 3-9g

Mo Yao (Resina Myrrhae)

Nature & flavor: Bitter, neutral
Channels entered: Heart, liver, spleen
Functions:
1. Quickens the blood and dispels stasis
2. Disperses swelling and alleviates pain
Dosage: 3-12g

Wang Bu Liu Xing (Semen Vaccariae Segetalis)

Nature & flavor: Bitter, neutral
Channels entered: Liver, stomach
Functions:
1. Quickens the blood and frees the flow of the channels
2. Frees the flow of the breasts (and/or milk)
3. Disperses swelling (in the breasts and/or testicles)
Dosage: 3-9g

Yu Jin (Tuber Curcumae)

Nature & flavor: Acrid, bitter, cool
Channels entered: Heart, lung, liver
Functions:
1. Quickens the blood and breaks stasis
2. Moves the qi
3. Clears the heart and cools the blood
4. Frees the flow of the gallbladder and abates jaundice
Dosage: 4.5-9g

Yan Hu Suo (Rhizoma Corydalis Yanhusuo)

Nature & flavor: Acrid, bitter, warm
Channels entered: Heart, liver, lung, stomach
Functions:
1. Quickens the blood and alleviates pain
2. Moves the qi and alleviates pain
Dosage: 4.5-12g

Wu Ling Zhi (Excrementum Trogopterori Seu Pteromi)

Nature & flavor: Bitter, sweet, warm
Channels entered: Liver, spleen
Functions:
1. Dispels stasis and alleviates pain
2. Transforms stasis and stops bleeding
Dosage: 3-9g

Chuan Shan Jia (Squama Manitis Pentadactylis)

Nature & flavor: Salty, cool
Channels entered: Liver, stomach
Functions:
1. Dispels stasis, frees the flow of the breasts (and/or milk), and frees the flow of menstruation
2. Disperses swelling and promotes the discharge of pus
3. Dispels wind and eliminates dampness from the channels
Dosage: 3-9g

Lu Lu Tong (Fructus Liquidambaris Taiwaniae)

Nature & flavor: Bitter, neutral
Channels entered: Liver, stomach
Functions:
1. Promotes the movement of qi and blood, opens the middle and frees the flow of the channels
2. Disinhibits urination and disperses swelling
Dosage: 3-9g

Stop-bleeding medicinals

Ai Ye (Folium Artemisiae Argyii)

Nature & flavor: Bitter, acrid, warm
Channels entered: Spleen, liver, kidney
Functions:
1. Warms the uterus and stops bleeding
2. Warms the uterus and quiets the fetus
3. Scatters cold and alleviates pain
Dosage: 3-9g

San Qi (Radix Notoginseng)

Nature & flavor: Sweet, slightly bitter, warm
Channels entered: Liver, stomach, large intestine
Functions:
1. Stops bleeding and transforms stasis
2. Disperses swelling and alleviates pain
Dosage: 3-9g

Pu Huang (Pollen Typhae)

Nature & flavor: Sweet, acrid, neutral
Channels entered: Liver, heart, spleen
Functions:
1. Stops bleeding
2. Quickens the blood and dispels stasis
Dosage: 4.5-12g

Di Yu (Radix Sanguisorbae Officinalis)

Nature & flavor: Bitter, sour, slightly cold
Channels entered: Liver, large intestine, stomach
Functions:
1. Cools the blood and stops bleeding
2. Clears heat and generates the flesh
Dosage: 6-15g

Ce Bai Ye (Cacumen Biotae Orientalis)

Nature & flavor: Bitter, astringent, slightly cold
Channels entered: Heart, liver, large intestine
Functions:
1. Cools the blood and stops bleeding
2. Stops coughing and expels phlegm
Dosage: 6-15g

Xue Yu Tan (Crinis Carbonisatus)

Nature & flavor: Bitter, neutral
Channels entered: Heart, liver, kidney
Functions:
1. Stops bleeding and secures leakage
2. Disinhibits urination and frees the flow of strangury
Dosage: 1.5-9g

Heavy, settling, spirit-quieting medicinals

Mu Li (Concha Ostreae)

Nature & flavor: Salty, astringent, cool
Channels entered: Liver, kidney
Functions:
1. Settles and quiets the spirit
2. Constrains yin and subdues yang
3. Prevents leakage of fluids
4. Softens the hard and scatters nodulation
5. Absorbs acid and alleviates pain
Dosage: 15-30g

Long Gu (Os Draconis)

Nature & flavor: Sweet, astringent, neutral
Channels entered: Heart, kidney, liver
Functions:
1. Settles and quiets the spirit
2. Settles the liver and subdues yang
3. Prevents leakage of fluids
Dosage: 15-30g

Heart-nourishing, spirit-quieting medicinals

Suan Zao Ren (Semen Zizyphi Spinosae)

Nature & flavor: Sweet, neutral
Channels entered: Gallbladder, heart, liver, spleen
Functions:
1. Nourishes heart yin, supplements liver blood, and quiets the spirit
2. Stops sweating
Dosage: 9-18g

Bai Zi Ren (Semen Biotae Orientalis)

Nature & flavor: Sweet, neutral
Channels entered: Heart, kidney, large intestine, spleen
Functions:
1. Nourishes the heart and quiets the spirit
2. Moistens the intestines and frees the flow of the stools
Dosage: 6-18g

Yuan Zhi (Radix Polygalae Tenuifoliae)

Nature & flavor: Bitter, acrid, slightly warm
Channels entered: Heart, lung
Functions:
1. Quiets the heart and calms the spirit
2. Expels phlegm and opens the orifices
3. Expels phlegm from the lungs
Dosage: 3-9g

Medicinals that abduct food & disperse stagnation

Shan Zha (Fructus Crataegi)
Nature & flavor: Sour, sweet, slightly warm
Channels entered: Liver, spleen, stomach
Functions:
1. Disperses food and abducts stagnation
2. Transforms stasis and disperses accumulations
3. Stops diarrhea
4. Reduces blood pressure
Dosage: 9-15g

Mai Ya (Fructus Germinatus Hordei Vulgaris)

Nature & flavor: Sweet, neutral
Channels entered: Liver, spleen, stomach
Functions:
1. Disperses food and fortifies the stomach
2. Stems lactation
3. Courses the liver and rectifies the qi
Dosage: 6-15g

Gu Ya (Fructus Germinatus Oryzae Sativae)

Nature & flavor: Sweet, neutral
Channels entered: Spleen, stomach
Functions: Disperses food and fortifies the stomach
Dosage: 9-15g

Shen Qu (Massa Medica Fermentata)

Nature & flavor: Sweet, acrid, warm
Channels entered: Spleen, stomach
Functions: Disperses food and harmonizes the stomach
Dosage: 6-15g

Wind-extinguishing medicinals

Tian Ma (Rhizoma Gastrodiae Elatae)

Nature & flavor: Sweet, neutral
Channels entered: Liver
Functions:
1. Settles the liver and extinguishes wind
2. Extinguishes wind, resolves tetany, and alleviates pain
3. Frees the flow of impediment and alleviates pain
Dosage: 3-9g

Medicinals that stop coughing & level panting

Kuan Dong Hua (Flos Tussilaginis Farfarae)

Nature & flavor: Acrid, warm
Channels entered: Lung
Functions: Downbears counterflow and stops coughing
Dosage: 4.5-9g

Xing Ren (Semen Pruni Armeniacae)

Nature & flavor: Bitter, slightly warm, slightly toxic
Channels entered: Large intestine, lung
Functions:
1. Stops coughing and levels panting
2. Moistens the intestines and frees the flow of the stools
Dosage: 3-9g

Worm-killing medicinals

Bing Lang (Semen Arecae Catechu)

Nature & flavor: Acrid, bitter, warm
Channels entered: Large intestine, stomach
Functions:
1. Kills worms
2. Moves the qi, disperses accumulations, and abducts stagnation
3. Moves the qi and disinhibits urination
Dosage: 6-12g

General Index

Formula Index

Formula Index

OTHER BOOKS ON CHINESE MEDICINE AVAILABLE FROM:
BLUE POPPY PRESS

5441 Western, Suite 2, Boulder, CO 80301
For ordering 1-800-487-9296 PH. 303-447-8372 FAX 303-245-8362
Email: info@bluepoppy.com Website: www.bluepoppy.com

ACUPOINT POCKET REFERENCE
by Bob Flaws
ISBN 0-936185-93-7

ACUPUNCTURE & IVF
by Lifang Liang
ISBN 0-891845-24-1

ACUPUNCTURE AND MOXIBUSTION
FORMULAS & TREATMENTS
by Cheng Dan-an, trans. by Wu Ming
ISBN 0-936185-68-6

ACUPUNCTURE PHYSICAL MEDICINE:
An Acupuncture Touchpoint Approach to the
Treatment of Chronic Pain, Fatigue, and
Stress Disorders
by Mark Seem
ISBN 1-891845-13-6

AGING & BLOOD STASIS:
A New Approach to TCM Geriatrics
by Yan De-xin
ISBN 0-936185-63-5

BETTER BREAST HEALTH NATURALLY
with CHINESE MEDICINE
by Honora Lee Wolfe & Bob Flaws
ISBN 0-936185-90-2

THE BOOK OF JOOK:
Chinese Medicinal Porridges
by BobFlaws
ISBN 0-936185-60-0

CHANNEL DIVERGENCES:
Deeper Pathways of the Web
by Miki Shima and Charles Chase
ISBN 1-891845-15-2

CHINESE MEDICAL PALMISTRY:
Your Health in Your Hand
by Zong Xiao-fan & Gary Liscum
ISBN 0-936185-64-3

CHINESE MEDICAL PSYCHIATRY
A Textbook and Clinical Manual
by Bob Flaws and James Lake, MD
ISBN 1-845891-17-9

CHINESE MEDICINAL TEAS:
Simple, Proven, Folk Formulas for
Common Diseases & Promoting Health
by Zong Xiao-fan & Gary Liscum
ISBN 0-936185-76-7

CHINESE MEDICINAL WINES & ELIXIRS
by Bob Flaws
ISBN 0-936185-58-9

CHINESE PEDIATRIC MASSAGE THERAPY:
A Parent's & Practitioner's Guide to the
Prevention & Treatment of Childhood Illness
by Fan Ya-li
ISBN 0-936185-54-6

CHINESE SELF-MASSAGE THERAPY:
The Easy Way to Health
by Fan Ya-li
ISBN 0-936185-74-0

CLASSIC OF DIFFICULTIES: A Translation of
the Nan Jing
translation by Bob Flaws
ISBN 1-891845-07-1

CLINICAL NEPHROLOGY
IN CHINESE MEDICINE
by Wei Li & David Frierman,
with Ben Luna & Bob Flaws
ISBN 1-891845-23-3

CONTROLLING DIABETES NATURALLY
WITH CHINESE MEDICINE
by Lynn Kuchinski
ISBN 0-936185-06-3

CURING ARTHRITIS NATURALLY WITH
CHINESE MEDICINE
by Douglas Frank & Bob Flaws
ISBN 0-936185-87-2

CURING DEPRESSION NATURALLY WITH
CHINESE MEDICINE
by Rosa Schnyer & Bob Flaws
ISBN 0-936185-94-5

CURING FIBROMYALGIA NATURALLY
WITH CHINESE MEDICINE
by Bob Flaws
ISBN 1-891845-09-8

CURING HAY FEVER NATURALLY WITH
CHINESE MEDICINE
by Bob Flaws
ISBN 0-936185-91-0

CURING HEADACHES NATURALLY WITH
CHINESE MEDICINE
by Bob Flaws
ISBN 0-936185-95-3

CURING IBS NATURALLY WITH CHINESE
MEDICINE
by Jane Bean Oberski
ISBN 1-891845-11-X

CURING INSOMNIA NATURALLY WITH
CHINESE MEDICINE
by Bob Flaws
ISBN 0-936185-86-4

CURING PMS NATURALLY WITH
CHINESE MEDICINE
by Bob Flaws
ISBN 0-936185-85-6

THE DIVINE FARMER'S MATERIA MEDICA:
A Translation of the Shen Nong Ben Cao
translation by Yang Shou-zhong
ISBN 0-936185-96-1

THE DIVINELY RESPONDING CLASSIC:
A Translation of the Shen Ying Jing from
Zhen Jiu Da Cheng
trans. by Yang Shou-zhong & Liu Feng-ting
ISBN 0-936185-55-4

DUI YAO: THE ART OF COMBINING
CHINESE HERBAL MEDICINALS
by Philippe Sionneau
ISBN 0-936185-81-3

ENDOMETRIOSIS, INFERTILITY AND
TRADITIONAL CHINESE MEDICINE:
A Laywoman's Guide
by Bob Flaws
ISBN 0-936185-14-7

THE ESSENCE OF LIU FENG-WU'S
GYNECOLOGY
by Liu Feng-wu, translated by Yang Shou-zhong
ISBN 0-936185-88-0

EXTRA TREATISES BASED ON
INVESTIGATION & INQUIRY:
A Translation of Zhu Dan-xi's Ge Zhi Yu Lun
translation by Yang Shou-zhong
ISBN 0-936185-53-8

FIRE IN THE VALLEY: TCM Diagnosis &
Treatment of Vaginal Diseases
by Bob Flaws
ISBN 0-936185-25-2

FU QING-ZHU'S GYNECOLOGY
trans. by Yang Shou-zhong and Liu Da-wei
ISBN 0-936185-35-X

FULFILLING THE ESSENCE:
A Handbook of Traditional & Contemporary
Treatments for Female Infertility
by Bob Flaws
ISBN 0-936185-48-1

GOLDEN NEEDLE WANG LE-TING: A 20th
Century Master's Approach to Acupuncture
by Yu Hui-chan and Han Fu-ru, trans. by Shuai
Xue-zhong
ISBN 0-936185-789-3

A GUIDE TO GYNECOLOGY
by Ye Heng-yin, trans. by Bob Flaws and Shuai
Xue-zhong
ISBN 1-891845-19-5

A HANDBOOK OF CHINESE
HEMATOLOGY
by Simon Becker
ISBN 1-891845-16-0

A HANDBOOK OF MENSTRUAL
DISEASES IN CHINESE MEDICINE
by Bob Flaws
ISBN 0-936185-82-1

A HANDBOOK OF TCM PATTERNS
& TREATMENTS
by Bob Flaws & Daniel Finney
ISBN 0-936185-70-8

A HANDBOOK of TCM PEDIATRICS
by Bob Flaws
ISBN 0-936185-72-4

A HANDBOOK OF TRADITIONAL
CHINESE DERMATOLOGY
by Liang Jian-hui, trans. by Zhang Ting-liang &
Bob Flaws
ISBN 0-936185-07-4

A HANDBOOK OF TRADITIONAL
CHINESE GYNECOLOGY by Zhejiang College
of TCM, trans. by Zhang Ting-liang & Bob Flaws

ISBN 0-936185-06-6 (4th ed.)

THE HEART & ESSENCE OF DAN-XI'S
METHODS OF TREATMENT
by Xu Dan-xi, trans. by Yang Shou-zhong
ISBN 0-926185-49-X

THE HEART TRANSMISSION
OF MEDICINE
by Liu Yi-ren, trans. by Yang Shou-zhong
ISBN 0-936185-83-X

HIGHLIGHTS OF ANCIENT
ACUPUNCTURE PRESCRIPTIONS
trans. by Honora Lee Wolfe & Rose Crescenz
ISBN 0-936185-23-6

IMPERIAL SECRETS OF HEALTH
& LONGEVITY
by Bob Flaws
ISBN 0-936185-51-1

INSIGHTS OF A SENIOR
ACUPUNCTURIST
by Miriam Lee
ISBN 0-936185-33-3

INTRODUCTION TO THE USE OF
PROCESSED CHINESE MEDICINALS
by Philippe Sionneau
ISBN 0-936185-62-7

KEEPING YOUR CHILD HEALTHY WITH
CHINESE MEDICINE
by Bob Flaws
ISBN 0-936185-71-6

THE LAKESIDE MASTER'S
STUDY OF THE PULSE
by Li SHI-zhen; trans. by Bob Flaws
ISBN 1-891845-01-2

MANAGING MENOPAUSE NATURALLY
with Chinese Medicine
by Honora Lee Wolfe
ISBN 0-936185-98-8

MASTER HUA'S CLASSIC OF THE
CENTRAL VISCERA
by Hua Tuo, trans. by Yang Shou-zhong
ISBN 0-936185-43-0

MASTER TONG'S ACUPUNCTURE
by Miriam Lee
ISBN 0-936185-37-6

THE MEDICAL I CHING: Oracle of the
Healer Within
by Miki Shima
ISBN 0-936185-38-4

A NEW AMERICAN ACUPUNTURE
by Mark Seem
ISBN 0-936185-44-9

PATH OF PREGNANCY, VOL. I,
Gestational Disorders
by Bob Flaws
ISBN 0-936185-39-2

PATH OF PREGNANCY, Vol. II,
Postpartum Diseases
by Bob Flaws
ISBN 0-936185-42-2

POINTS FOR PROFIT
by Honora Wolfe, Eric Strand, Marilyn Allen
ISBN 1-891845-25-X

THE PULSE CLASSIC:
A Translation of the Mai Jing
by Wang Shu-he, trans. by Yang Shou-zhong
ISBN 0-936185-75-9

RECENT TCM RESEARCH FROM CHINA
by Bob Flaws and Charles Chase
ISBN 0-936185-56-2

THE SECRET OF CHINESE
PULSE DIAGNOSIS
by Bob Flaws
ISBN 0-936185-67-8

SHAOLIN SECRET FORMULAS for
Treatment of External Injuries
by De Chan, trans. by Zhang Ting-liang &
Bob Flaws
ISBN 0-936185-08-2

STATEMENTS OF FACT IN TRADITIONAL
CHINESE MEDICINE
by Bob Flaws
ISBN 0-936185-52-X

STICKING TO THE POINT 1:
A Rational Methodology for the Step by
Step Formulation & Administration of
an Acupuncture Treatment
by Bob Flaws
ISBN 0-936185-17-1

STICKING TO THE POINT 2:
A Study of Acupuncture & Moxibustion
Formulas and Strategies
by Bob Flaws
ISBN 0-936185-97-X

A STUDY OF DAOIST ACUPUNCTURE
by Liu Zheng-cai
ISBN 1-891845-08-X

THE SYSTEMATIC CLASSIC OF
ACUPUNCTURE & MOXIBUSTION: A
Translation of the *Jia Yi Jing*
by Huang-fu Mi, trans. by Yang Shou-zhong &
Charles Chase
ISBN 0-936185-29-5

THE TAO OF HEALTHY EATING
ACCORDING TO CHINESE MEDICINE
by Bob Flaws
ISBN 0-936185-92-9

TEACH YOURSELF TO READ MODERN
MEDICAL CHINESE
by Bob Flaws
ISBN 0-936185-99-6

Li Dong-yaun's TREATISE ON THE SPLEEN
& STOMACH: A Translation of the Pi Wei
Lun
trans. by Yang Shou-zhong
ISBN 0-936185-41-4

THE TREATMENT OF CARDIOVASCULAR
DISEASES WITH CHINESE MEDICINE
by Simon Becker, Bob Flaws & Robert Casañas,
MD
ISBN 978-1-891845-27-6

THE TREATMENT OF DIABETES
MELLITUS WITH CHINESE MEDICINE
by Bob Flaws, Lynn Kuchinski & Robert
Casañas, MD
ISBN 1-891845-21-7

THE TREATMENT OF DISEASE IN TCM,
Vol. 1: Diseases of the Head & Face,
Including Mental & Emotional Disorders
by Philippe Sionneau & Lü Gang
ISBN 0-936185-69-4

THE TREATMENT OF DISEASE IN TCM,
Vol. II: Diseases of the Eyes, Ears,
Nose, & Throat
by Philippe Sionneau & Lü Gang
ISBN 0-936185-73-2

THE TREATMENT OF DISEASE, Vol. III:
Diseases of the Mouth, Lips, Tongue,
Teeth & Gums
by Philippe Sionneau & Lü Gang
ISBN 0-936185-79-1

THE TREATMENT OF DISEASE, Vol. IV:
Diseases of the Neck, Shoulders,
Back, & Limbs
by Philippe Sionneau & Lü Gang
ISBN 0-936185-89-9

THE TREATMENT OF DISEASE, Vol. V:
Diseases of the Chest & Abdomen
by Philippe Sionneau & Lü Gang
ISBN 1-891845-02-0

THE TREATMENT OF DISEASE, Vol. VI:
Diseases of the Urogential System
& Proctology
by Philippe Sionneau & Lü Gang
ISBN 1-891845-05-5

THE TREATMENT OF DISEASE, Vol. VII:
General Symptoms
by Philippe Sionneau & Lü Gang
ISBN 1-891845-14-4

THE TREATMENT OF EXTERNAL
DISEASES WITH ACUPUNCTURE
& MOXIBUSTION
by Yan Cui-lan and Zhu Yun-long, trans. by Yang
Shou-zhong
ISBN 0-936185-80-5

THE TREATMENT OF MODERN
WESTERN MEDICAL DISEASES
WITH CHINESE MEDICINE
by Bob Flaws & Philippe Sionneau
ISBN 1-891845-20-9

70 ESSENTIAL CHINESE
HERBAL FORMULAS
by Bob Flaws
ISBN 0-936185-59-7

160 ESSENTIAL CHINESE HERBAL
PATENT MEDICINES
by Bob Flaws
ISBN 1-891945-12-8

230 ESSENTIAL CHINESE MEDICINALS
by Bob Flaws
ISBN 1-891845-03-9

630 QUESTIONS & ANSWERS ABOUT
CHINESE HERBAL MEDICINE:
A Workbook & Study Guide
by Bob Flaws
ISBN 1-891845-04-7

750 QUESTIONS & ANSWERS ABOUT
ACUPUNCTURE
Exam Preparation & Study Guide
by Fred Jennes
ISBN 1-891845-22-5